THIRD EDITION
# MEDICALLY IMPORTANT FUNGI
## A GUIDE TO IDENTIFICATION

THIRD EDITION

# MEDICALLY IMPORTANT FUNGI

## A GUIDE TO IDENTIFICATION

**DAVISE H. LARONE**
Ph.D., SM(AAM), MT(ASCP)
Diplomate, American Board of
Medical Microbiology

Mycology Resource Center
Clinical Microbiology Service
Columbia Presbyterian Medical Center
New York, New York

Illustrated by the author

**ASM Press**
Washington, D.C.

Copyright © 1976, 1987, 1995  American Society for Microbiology
1325 Massachusetts Ave., N.W.
Washington, DC 20005

**Library of Congress Cataloging-in-Publication Data**

Medically important fungi: a guide to identification / by Davise H. Larone. — 3rd ed.
   p.    cm.
    Rev. ed. of: Medically important fungi / Davise H. Larone. 2nd ed. c1987.
    Includes bibliographical references and index.
    ISBN 1-55581-091-8
    1. Pathogenic fungi—Identification.  2. Fungi—Cultures and culture media.
  3. Medical mycology.  I. Larone, Davise Honig, 1939–   . II. Larone, Davise Honig,
  1939–    Medically important fungi.
    [DNLM: 1. Fungi—chemistry.   QW 25M4895 1995]
QR245.L37   1995
616'.015—dc20
DNLM/DLC
for Library of Congress
                                       94–40202
                                         CIP

Current printing (last digit)
10  9  8  7  6  5  4  3

Dedicated with love
to
Ronit,
Frank,
and
in memory of John D. Lawrence

# Contents

# List of Tables

# Preface to the Third Edition

With the third edition of *Medically Important Fungi: a Guide to Identification*, I am as committed as ever to making and keeping this book a truly useful tool for technical staffs, medical technology students, pathology residents, and others who attempt to identify fungi in the clinical mycology laboratory.

With the increase in numbers and types of immunocompromised individuals predisposed to fungal infection, our field is growing in importance, scope, and complexity. Organisms that were in the past relatively unknown or considered harmless saprophytes are today encountered as etiologic agents of infection. Organisms that were once thought to infect only specific sites, such as subcutaneous tissue, are now causing disease in other areas. To accommodate these developments, descriptions of 22 organisms have been added to this edition, and the detailed descriptions of the thermally monomorphic molds are grouped according to culture characteristics rather than by the expected site of infection (with the exception of the dermatophytes). An introductory page with a brief discussion and overview of the organisms that follow now precedes each group of fungi. The section on dematiaceous (black) fungi has been expanded to include more tables to help differentiate similar organisms. Five laboratory procedures and two staining methods have been inserted. Nomenclature and information for each organism have been updated.

The most dramatic modification to this edition is the incorporation of photomicrographs to accompany the line drawings. The two forms of illustration are meant not to duplicate but to complement one another. Photomicrographs of organisms as seen on culture are included with the detailed descriptions, but photomicrographs are not yet included in the section on direct microscopic examination; that is planned for the next edition. Referrals for further information on each organism have been updated and include only books that are presently in print; this means that some dear old favorites had to be deleted.

Users of previous editions will certainly notice the new style of binding. It is hoped that this will sustain the book through heavy routine laboratory usage and hold it intact much longer than was common with earlier editions.

No publication of this sort is accomplished without a great deal of help from others. I am continually moved by the generosity of my colleagues who so willingly contributed information, suggestions, organisms, and precious photomicrographs. My thanks go to Joan Barenfanger, Mary Clancy, Chet Cooper, Dennis Dixon, Morris Gordon, Jim Harris, Kevin Hazen, Geoffrey Land, Evelyn Koestenblatt, Vincent LaBombardi, Michael McGinnis, Bill Merz, Arvind Padhye, Michael Rinaldi, Mark Romagnoli, Glenn Roberts, Stanley Rosenthal, Lynne Sigler, Richard Summerbell, and, last (in alphabetical order only), Irene Weitzman. I am particularly indebted to Ira Salkin who was always ready to discuss, instruct, and advise whenever I phoned.

There are many others to whom I owe gratitude: the staff of my laboratory at Lenox Hill Hospital and staffs of many other labs who have expressed their need and appreciation for the book and have given me helpful feedback to improve each edition; Rose Marie Spitaleri and George Tanis for assistance in medical photography; Brent Dorsett for his computer wizardry in enlarging and clarifying some seemingly unsalvageable photomicrographs; Joseph O'Brien for word processing; the book publishing team at ASM Press for their enthusiasm, talent, and hard work; and especially Frank Anderson, without whose computer assistance and moral support the manuscript would have been much more difficult to prepare.

*New York City*
*September 1994*

# Preface to the First Edition

More than ever, clinical laboratory personnel with limited experience in mycology must culture and identify fungi isolated from clinical specimens. Even after attending a course in the subject, technologists often need guidance in identifying the great variety of organisms encountered in the lab. With the advent of proficiency testing by local and national organizations, technologists have a need and opportunity to practice and increase their skills in the medical mycology laboratory.

Most classic texts, though rich in information, are arranged according to the clinical description of the infection; the textual discussion of any particular fungus can be located only from the index or table of contents. Since the technologist doesn't know the name of an unidentified fungus and usually has little or no knowledge of the clinical picture, these texts are at best difficult to use effectively. The unfortunate result is the all-too-common practice of flipping through an entire mycology textbook in search of a picture that resembles the organism under examination. Such a practice may make the more accomplished mycologist's hair stand on end, but it is a fact to be acknowledged.

This guide is not meant to compete with these large texts, but to complement them. The material here is so arranged that the technician can systematically reach a possible identification knowing only the macro- and microscopic morphology of an isolated organism. Reference can then be made to one of the classic texts for confirmation and detailed information.

Many possible variants of organisms are found under several categories of morphology and pigment. The outstanding characteristics are listed on the page(s) apportioned to each organism, and references are suggested for further information and confirmation (see How to Use the Guide).

*Medically Important Fungi* avoids the jargon so commonly and confusingly used in most mycology books. Drawings are used wherever possible to illustrate organisms described in the text. To ensure clarity, a glossary of terms is included, as well as a section on laboratory techniques for observing proper morphology. Another section includes use of the various media, stains, and tests mentioned in the book.

The actinomycetes, although now known to be bacteria rather than fungi, are included because they are frequently handled in the mycology section of the clinical laboratory.

It is believed that this guide will enable students and medical technologists to culture and identify fungi with greater ease and competency and in so doing to develop an appreciation of the truly beautiful microscopic forms encountered.

I wish to acknowledge with gratitude the encouragement and advice received from my co-workers at Lenox Hill Hospital, and Dr. Norman Goodman, Mr. Gerald Krefetz, Mr. Bill Rosenzweig, Ms. Eve Rothenberg, Dr. Guenther Stotzky, Mr. Martin Weisburd, Dr. Irene Weitzman and Dr. Marion E. Wilson.

*New York*
*December 1975*

# How to Use the Guide

Before beginning to use the guide, several points should be understood.

Fungi often appear differently in living hosts than they do in cultures. Chapter 1 is designed as a guide for preliminary identification of fungi seen on direct microscopic examination of clinical specimens.

In chapters 2 through 6, the descriptions of the macroscopic and microscopic morphologies of the cultured fungi pertain to those on Sabouraud dextrose agar unless otherwise specified.

Many molds begin as white mycelial growths, and coloration occurs at the time of conidiation or sporulation. Hence, organisms are listed under their most likely color(s) at maturity, when the typical microscopic reproductive formations are more readily observed.

This book is a *guide to identification*. The standard texts should be used for additional information concerning clinical disease, history, ecology, immunology, and therapy.

Instructions for general procedures prior to identification, i.e., collection of specimens, direct microscopic preparations, primary isolation, slide cultures, special tests, and the like, are given in chapter

7. Staining methods are described in chapter 8; preparation and use of media are explained in chapter 9.

Once the organism has been properly collected, cultured, isolated, and observed microscopically, use of the guide is quite simple:

1. Note the morphology of the unknown fungus.
   a. Is it a filamentous bacterium, yeastlike, thermally dimorphic, or a thermally monomorphic mold?
   b. Record color of surface and reverse (underside) of colony.
2. Using the initial "Guide to the Identification of Fungi in Culture" on p. 18, refer to a page that shows drawings of the microscopic morphology of organisms having the appropriate macroscopic appearance. Here one may see either the exact organism under examination or several possibilities.
3. Proceed to the page written in parentheses next to the likely organism(s) and find more detailed information including pathogenicity, rate of growth, colony morphology, an enlarged drawing of the microscopic appearance, a photomicrograph, tests or facts that may help to differentiate between extremely similar organisms, and references for additional information.
4. Ordinarily the identification will be quite certain. If, however, any doubt remains, the organism should be sent to a reference laboratory for confirmation of identification as discussed in the following section.

# Use of Reference Laboratories

Rare or atypical fungi can be difficult to identify even for a very experienced microbiologist or medical technologist. After a possible identification of an isolated organism is reached, confirmation is often necessary.

When the identification of an isolated fungus is dubious or when the fungus appears to be one that the laboratory worker has never before encountered, a reliable reference laboratory should be asked to confirm the identification. Because of the toxicity of antifungal medications, it is especially important to confirm the identification of organisms suspected of causing systemic mycoses. Ordinarily, the state health department acts as a reference laboratory; in some localities the city department of health or other local laboratories supply the service.

Cultures sent to reference laboratories should be pure, young, and actively growing on agar slants. Petri plates should not be used. For details on the labeling, mailing, and delivering of potentially pathogenic isolates, one should consult the reference laboratory for specific requirements and comply with the *Interstate Shipment of Etiologic Agents* code:

1. The tube containing the slanted culture must be labeled with organism identification and must be securely closed and watertight (waterproof tape seal is advisable). The culture tube is considered the primary container.
2. Place enough absorbent, nonparticulate material at the top, bottom, and sides of the culture tube to absorb the entire volume of the culture in case of breakage or leakage.
3. Insert the wrapped culture tube into a secondary durable, watertight container (usually a metal cylinder). Several culture tubes may be placed in a single secondary container, but the total contents cannot exceed 50 ml.
4. Place the secondary container(s) in an outer shipping container constructed of cardboard, wood, metal, or other material of equivalent strength; cardboard or metal screw-cap mailing tubes are most commonly used.
5. Affix the address label to the outer shipping container (the return address should contain the sender's telephone number); include an official "Etiologic Agent" label (shown below), which is available from the Centers for Disease Control and Prevention (CDC) and label manufacturers.
6. If the organism being transported is suspected of being *Coccidioides immitis, Histoplasma capsulatum,* or another systemic pathogen, it must be shipped in a manner that provides for sending notification of receipt back to the sender. If receipt is not confirmed within 5 days following anticipated delivery, the sender must notify the CDC.

For an exceptionally clear illustration of proper packaging see *Biosafety in Microbiological and Biomedical Laboratories*, 3rd ed., U.S. Department of Health and Human Services Publication no. (CDC) 93-8395 [Atlanta: CDC, 1993], p. 149.

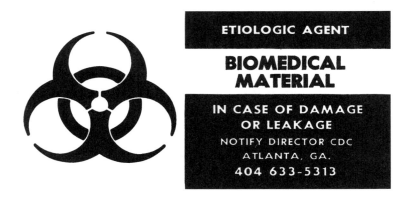

ETIOLOGIC AGENT

**BIOMEDICAL MATERIAL**

IN CASE OF DAMAGE OR LEAKAGE
NOTIFY DIRECTOR CDC
ATLANTA, GA.
404 633-5313

# Safety Precautions

Since many fungi produce conidia or spores that easily become airborne, precautions are essential to prevent contamination of the laboratory environment and infection of the personnel.

A suitable biological safety cabinet (class 1 or 2) should be used when dealing with molds. Yeast cultures can be handled in the same manner that bacterial cultures are routinely handled.

Care must be taken not to spatter infectious material by careless flaming of wire needles or loops. Bacti-Cinerators are recommended to avoid this hazard. Sterile, disposable implements may be the best solution, by eliminating the need to flame.

Tubed slants of media are safer to handle than plates. If plates are used, shrink seals should be employed. Petri plates should NEVER be used if *Coccidioides immitis* is suspected or if a culture is to be mailed or otherwise transported to another laboratory.

A wet preparation should be made of all molds before setting up a slide culture; do NOT set up slide cultures of isolates that may be *Histoplasma, Blastomyces, Coccidioides,* or *Paracoccidioides* spp. or *Xylohypha bantiana.*

Decant supernatants into containers of disinfectant.

All contaminated materials must be autoclaved before discarding.

Hands should be thoroughly washed with a disinfectant soap after handling mycology cultures.

The work area should be cleaned with disinfectant at least daily.

Laboratory coats should be worn at all times in the work area.

Do not mouth pipet.

There should be no smoking, drinking, eating, gum chewing, application of cosmetics, or insertion of contact lenses in the laboratory.

NEVER sniff a fungal culture to determine whether it has an odor.

# Guides

# Guide to Interpretation of Direct Microscopic Examination of Clinical Specimens

1

Specimens submitted to the mycology laboratory from skin, tissue, normally sterile body fluids, and patients strongly suspected of having a fungal infection should be examined microscopically for the presence of fungal elements. This examination is important for several reasons.

It may provide the physician with a rapid diagnosis and information regarding the possible need for treatment.

It is helpful in determining the significance of the organism that will later be definitively identified on culture. If the organism is one that is only sometimes pathogenic and was seen on the direct microscopic examination in appreciable numbers it is more likely that it is involved in a disease process and not merely present as a contaminant. In cases of suspected candidiasis, pseudohyphae invading tissue indicate infection as opposed to colonization.

Observation of unique fungal elements may indicate the need for special media, specimens from other sites, and/or serological tests.

Table 1.1 is meant to aid mycology personnel in reading direct smears and wet preps as well as tissue sections. The drawing and written description of the microscopic morphology are to be considered together. The sites of infection are listed in approximate order of frequency, and the interpretation states the disease suggested along with the etiologic agent(s). In some cases, the direct microscopic examination yields a relatively certain identification (yet presumptive, to be confirmed by culture) of the organism; in many other instances, culture is the only means of identification.

Methods for direct microscopic examination of specimens are outlined in chapter 7 (pp. 212–214). Staining methods are described in chapter 8 (pp. 225–232). Of the special stains for fungi, Gomori's methenamine silver nitrate has long been considered by many to be the most useful. It can be used on smears as well as tissue and is routinely performed in histology laboratories; a simplified method is provided on p. 228. A newer and very successful stain for fungi is calcofluor white (p. 227). Other commonly used tissue stains mentioned in Table 1.1 are hematoxylin and eosin, Gridley fungus, and periodic acid-Schiff.

Those who lack confidence in reading tissue sections for fungal infections because of unfamiliarity with the background cellular reaction are referred to the clear and concise review of inflammatory tissue reactions by Koneman and Roberts (1991).

For further information and excellent photomicrographs of fungi in tissue, see Chandler and Watts (1987).

**TABLE 1.1** Characteristic features of fungi and actinomycetes seen on direct examination of clinical specimens[a]

| Observation | Description | Sites of infection | Interpretation and etiologic agent(s) |
|---|---|---|---|
| | Granules from abscess or draining sinus tracts are cream to white "sulfur granules" (30–3,000 μm or more in diameter) that, when crushed, appear as opaque masses with peripheral, gelatinous, club-shaped bodies. Granules contain numerous delicate (less than 1 μm diameter), branched filaments that are gram positive and non-acid fast; they stain with GMS and Giemsa stains, but not with H&E, GF, and PAS. | Facial-neck area<br>Lung<br>Thoracic cavity<br>Abdominal cavity<br>Multiple systemic sites | ACTINOMYCOSIS<br>*Actinomyces israelii*<br>Other *Actinomyces* spp. |
| | Granules (from subcutaneous tissues) 2.5–2,000 μm or more in diameter. | Subcutaneous tissue<br>Skin | ACTINOMYCOTIC OR EUMYCOTIC MYCETOMA |
| | Granule (white, yellow, or red) composed of narrow (0.5–1 μm in diameter) intertwined filaments with coccoid and bacillary forms. *Nocardia* spp. are usually at least partially acid fast, and *Actinomadura* spp. are not acid fast. All are gram positive and stain well with GMS and Giemsa stains but not with H&E, GF, and PAS. | Subcutaneous tissue<br>Skin | ACTINOMYCOTIC MYCETOMA<br>*Nocardia* spp.<br>*Actinomadura* spp.<br>*Streptomyces* spp. |
| | Granules (white, yellow, brown, or black) contain hyphae (2–6 μm in diameter) and often numerous chlamydospores and swollen cells, especially at the periphery of the granule. | Subcutaneous tissue<br>Skin | EUMYCOTIC MYCETOMA<br>*Pseudallescheria boydii*<br>*Madurella* spp.<br>*Exophiala jeanselmei*<br>*Acremonium* spp.<br>*Curvularia* spp.<br>Other molds, occasionally |

[a]For further information and excellent photomicrographs of fungi as they appear in clinical specimens, see Chandler and Watts (1987). Abbreviations: GMS, Gomori methenamine silver; H&E, hematoxylin and eosin; GF, Gridley fungus stain; PAS, periodic acid-Schiff.

**TABLE 1.1** Characteristic features of fungi and actinomycetes seen on direct examination of clinical specimens[a] *(continued)*

| Observation | Description | Sites of infection | Interpretation and etiologic agent(s) |
|---|---|---|---|
| | Delicate, narrow (0.5–1.0 μm in diameter) filaments that tend to branch at right angles; frequently appear beaded or granular when Gram stained; coccobacillary elements may also form; stain best with GMS when the staining time in the silver nitrate solution is increased; characteristically partially acid fast. | Lung<br>Skin, subcutaneous tissue<br>Central nervous system<br>Multiple systemic sites | NOCARDIOSIS<br>*Nocardia asteroides*<br>*Nocardia brasiliensis*<br>*Nocardia otitidiscaviarum (caviae)* |
| | Septate hyphae (3–6 μm in diameter) have dichotomous branching (each branch is approximately equal in width to the originating stem) at 45° angles. In chronic lesions, short, distorted hyphae may be as wide as 12 μm. Conidial heads and/or conidia may occasionally be seen; conidia may appear indented and crescent shaped and may stain unevenly with GMS. Many other fungi appear similar to the aspergilli in tissue or clinical specimens. However, zygomycetes have hyphae that are broader (almost nonseptate), often appear collapsed and twisted, and usually stain lighter with GMS; *Candida* spp., in addition to hyphae, form pseudohyphae and budding yeast cells. Hyphae of other opportunistic molds such as *Fusarium* spp. and *Pseudallescheria boydii* may be indistinguishable from those of *Aspergillus* spp. in tissue (but *P. boydii* usually has hyphae that are narrower and branch at broader angles). | Lung<br>Urine<br>Nasal sinus<br>Ear, eye<br>Skin, mucous membranes<br>Multiple systemic sites | ASPERGILLOSIS<br>*Aspergillus fumigatus*<br>Other *Aspergillus* spp. |
| | Hyphae broad (3–25 μm in diameter; average, 12 μm), infrequently septate, with nonparallel sides; branching nondichotomous, irregular, sometimes at right angles. Hyphae may appear distorted with swollen cells or compressed, twisted, and folded. Thick-walled chlamydospores (15–30 μm in diameter) may form. The special fungus stains (GMS, GF, PAS) generally do not color the zygomycetes as deeply as they do other fungi. | Lung<br>Nasal sinus<br>Brain<br>Eye<br>Skin, mucous membranes<br>Multiple systemic sites | ZYGOMYCOSIS<br>*Absidia corymbifera*<br>*Rhizopus* spp.<br>*Mucor* spp.<br>*Rhizomucor pusillus*<br>*Apophysomyces elegans*<br>*Saksenaea vasiformis*<br>*Cunninghamella bertholletiae*<br>*Basidiobolus* spp. (subcutaneous)<br>*Conidiobolus* spp. (subcutaneous) |

| | Description | Site | Disease and etiologic agents |
|---|---|---|---|
| | Colorless, branched, septate hyphae that may break up into chains of arthroconidia. Other conidia do not form in tissue. When hair is infected, arthroconidia may form on the outside of the hair (ectothrix type of invasion) or inside the hair (endothrix type). Hyphae can be found within the hair in both types. | Skin<br>Hair<br>Nails | DERMATOPHYTOSES (tinea, ringworm)<br>*Microsporum* spp.<br>*Trichophyton* spp.<br>*Epidermophyton floccosum* |
| | Darkly pigmented, branched, septate hyphae (1.5–3.0 µm in diameter) and sometimes elongated budding cells (1.5–5.0 µm in diameter) and chlamydoconidia. | Palm of hand<br>Other skin surfaces occasionally | TINEA NIGRA<br>*Phaeoannellomyces werneckii* |
| | Short, slightly curved, septate hyphal elements (2.5–4.0 µm in diameter) that form short chains; clusters of oval to round thick-walled cells (3–8 µm in diameter) that produce buds through small phialidic collarettes. The etiologic agent, *M. furfur*, will only grow on mycologic media that have been overlaid with 1–2 ml of sterile olive oil or supplemented with a long-chain fatty acid. | Skin<br>Systemic (catheter associated) | TINEA VERSICOLOR<br>*Malassezia furfur* |
| | Brown-pigmented, branched or unbranched, septate hyphae (2–6 µm in diameter). Hyphae are often constricted at thick, prominent, close septations and sometimes contain large, thick-walled, chlamydoconidium-like structures singly or in chains. Dark budding yeastlike forms may also occur. | Skin, subcutaneous tissue<br>Brain (*X. bantiana*)<br>Lung and other organs (rare) | PHAEOHYPHOMYCOSIS<br>*Exophiala jeanselmei*<br>*Wangiella dermatitidis*<br>*Bipolaris* spp.<br>*Xylohypha bantiana*<br>Other dematiaceous fungi |

[a] For further information and excellent photomicrographs of fungi as they appear in clinical specimens, see Chandler and Watts (1987). Abbreviations: GMS, Gomori methenamine silver; H&E, hematoxylin and eosin; GF, Gridley fungus stain; PAS, periodic acid-Schiff.

**TABLE 1.1** Characteristic features of fungi and actinomycetes seen on direct examination of clinical specimens[a] (continued)

| Observation | Description | Sites of infection | Interpretation and etiologic agent(s) |
|---|---|---|---|
| | Brown-pigmented, round to polyhedral, thick-walled sclerotic bodies (5–12 μm in diameter), having horizontal and/or vertical septations. Brown-pigmented, branched, distorted, septate hyphae (3–8 μm in diameter) may also be present. | Skin, subcutaneous tissue Systemic sites (very rare) | CHROMOBLASTOMYCOSIS *Fonsecaea pedrosoi* *Fonsecaea compacta* *Phialophora verrucosa* *Cladosporium carrioni* |
| | Yeastlike cells of various sizes and shapes; round to oval (2–6 μm in diameter) or characteristically elongated "cigar bodies" (2 × 3 to 3 × 10 μm). Buds form on a narrow base. In most cases, very few organisms are found on direct examination of clinical materials; fluorescent-antibody staining is helpful in observing the organism on direct preparations but is not readily available in most laboratories. | Skin, subcutaneous tissue Systemic sites (rare) | SPOROTRICHOSIS *Sporothrix schenckii* |
| | Small yeast cells (2–4 μm in diameter) with macrophages; yeast cells usually ovoid, with budding on a narrow base at the smaller end. In Giemsa- or Wright-stained preparations, a pale blue ring (the fungus cell wall) surrounds the darker blue protoplasm, and the cytoplasm retracts from the wall, often giving the false impression of a capsule; the chromatin stains dark violet and appears as a crescent-shaped mass within the protoplasm. The organism stains well and evenly with GMS or PAS. | Lung Blood, bone marrow Skin, mucous membranes Urine Multiple systemic sites | HISTOPLASMOSIS *Histoplasma capsulatum* |
| | Oval yeast cells (approximately 3 μm in diameter) within histiocytes, resembling *Histoplasma capsulatum*. Outside of histiocytes, yeast cells are up to 8 μm (sometimes curved), with a prominent central septum. The organism stains well with GMS or PAS (not H&E). | Blood, bone marrow Skin, mucous membranes Lung Lymph node Urine, stool Multiple systemic sites | PENICILLIOSIS *Penicillium marneffei* |

| | Description | Sites | Disease / Organism |
|---|---|---|---|
| | Yeastlike cells (3–30 μm in diameter; average, 7–15 μm), round to oval, with sharply defined cell walls that appear to be thick. Cells produce only one bud, which is distinctively attached to the parent cell by a very wide base (average, 4–5 μm). Budding in vivo is relatively infrequent. | Lung<br>Skin, mucous membranes<br>Urine<br>Multiple systemic sites | **BLASTOMYCOSIS**<br>*Blastomyces dermatitidis* |
| | Yeastlike cells, round to oval, large (5–60 μm in diameter); single and multiple buds are attached to the parent cell by narrow connections. Buds may be small and all approximately the same size or fairly large and of unequal sizes and shapes. | Lung<br>Skin, mucous membranes<br>Multiple systemic sites | **PARACOCCIDIOIDOMYCOSIS**<br>*Paracoccidioides brasiliensis* |
| | Branching septate hyphae, pseudohyphae, chains of budding cells, and individual round to oval budding yeast cells (blastoconidia, 3–5 μm in diameter). | Blood<br>Urine<br>Skin, nails<br>Mucous membranes<br>Multiple systemic sites | **CANDIDIASIS (CANDIDOSIS)**<br>*Candida albicans*<br>Other *Candida* spp. |
| | Budding yeast cells (2–20 μm in diameter) with thin dark walls. Capsules can be demonstrated by India ink in most clinical specimens; sputum or pus can be cleared with potassium hydroxide and heat and then mixed with India ink. Tissues stained with mucicarmine show the capsule as bright carmen red, often with a spiney or scalloped appearance; drying, fixing, and staining may cause the yeast cells to collapse or become crescent shaped. | Lung<br>Blood<br>Urine<br>Cerebrospinal fluid<br>Skin, mucous membranes<br>Multiple systemic sites | **CRYPTOCOCCOSIS**<br>*Cryptococcus neoformans* |

[a] For further information and excellent photomicrographs of fungi as they appear in clinical specimens, see Chandler and Watts (1987). Abbreviations: GMS, Gomori methenamine silver; H&E, hematoxylin and eosin; GF, Gridley fungus stain; PAS, periodic acid-Schiff.

**TABLE 1.1** Characteristic features of fungi and actinomycetes seen on direct examination of clinical specimens[a] (*continued*)

| Observation | Description | Sites of infection | Interpretation and etiologic agent(s) |
|---|---|---|---|
| | Nonbudding, round, ovoid, or collapsed crescent forms (3–5 μm in diameter). Cells often appear in small clusters on a thick foamy background. Cysts stain best with GMS and appear to have a dark area in the center. Toluidine blue O and calcofluor white are also used. Immunospecific stain is commercially available. | Lung<br>Multiple systemic sites | PNEUMOCYSTOSIS<br>*Pneumocystis carinii*[b] |
| | Round or oval sporangia (or spherules) ranging from 2–11 μm in diameter (*P. wickerhamii*) to 10–25 μm in diameter (*P. zopfii*). A sporangium contains 2–20 or more round, polyhedral, or cuboidal endospores. Size of the mother cells and differences in the numbers and morphologies of endospores help differentiate *Prototheca* from *Coccidioides* in direct preparations. | Skin<br>Subcutaneous tissue<br>Systemic sites (rare) | PROTOTHECOSIS<br>*Prototheca wickerhamii*<br>*Prototheca zopfii* |
| | Thick-walled, round spherules (10–80 μm or more in diameter); immature spherules occur as round cells with or without homogeneous contents; mature spherules contain many round endospores (2–5 μm in diameter). Fragmented or empty ruptured spherules are rare but sometimes observed in cavitary and necrotic lesions. | Lung<br>Mucous membranes<br>Skin<br>Urine<br>Blood<br>Multiple systemic sites | COCCIDIOIDOMYCOSIS<br>*Coccidioides immitis* |

RHINOSPORIDIOSIS
*Rhinosporidium seeberi*

Nasal mucosa
Mucosa of other body sites

Large, round sporangia (6–350 μm in diameter). Immature sporangia contain amorphous cytoplasm and a central nucleus. Mature sporangia may contain both immature and mature spores. Mature spores (7–9 μm in diameter) appear lobulated and contain globular bodies. The etiologic agent, *R. seeberi*, cannot be cultured; diagnosis depends on direct examination of nasal or other mucosal polyps.

ADIASPIROMYCOSIS
*Emmonsia parva var. crescens*

Lung

Large, round (150–300 μm in diameter) thick-walled (20–70 μm thick) adiospores. The interior usually appears empty, but some may contain faintly PAS-positive and eosinophilic granules (1–3 μm in diameter).

[a]For further information and excellent photomicrographs of fungi as they appear in clinical specimens, see Chandler and Watts (1987). Abbreviations: GMS, Gomori methenamine silver; H&E, hematoxylin and eosin; GF, Gridley fungus stain; PAS, periodic acid-Schiff.

[b]The taxonomic position of *Pneumocystis carinii* is controversial; phylogenically it appears to belong in the periphery of the kingdom *Fungi*.

# Guide to Identification of Fungi in Culture

# 2

*(continued)*

**Thermally Monomorphic Molds** (*continued*)

## FILAMENTOUS BACTERIA

Very thin (1 μm or less in diameter) branching filaments*
**Aerobic Actinomycetes**

*Nocardia* (p. **55**)

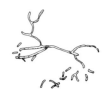

*Streptomyces* (p. **57**)

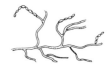

*Actinomadura* (p. **58**)

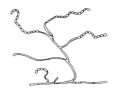

*Nocardiopsis* (p. **59**)

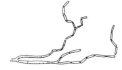

---

*Growth characteristics and biochemical tests must be utilized for identifications; these are summarized in Table 3.1 (p. 56).

# MONOMORPHIC YEASTS AND YEASTLIKE ORGANISMS

Yeastlike at 25–30°C and also at 35–37°C if growth occurs
**All rapid growers except** *Ustilago* **spp.**
**All WHITE, CREAM, or TAN except** *Rhodotorula* **and** *Sporobolomyces* **spp.**

Microscopic morphology on Cornmeal-Tween 80 agar (Dalmau plate)*

---

### Pseudohyphae with blastoconidia

*Candida albicans* (p. **63**)

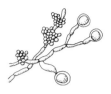

*Candida tropicalis* (p. **65**)

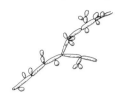

*Candida parapsilosis* (p. **68**)

*Candida lusitaniae* (p. **69**)

*Candida krusei* (p. **70**)

*Candida kefyr (pseudotropicalis)*
(p. **71**)

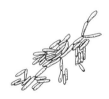

*Candida guilliermondii* (p. **72**)

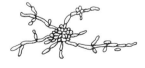

*Candida lipolytica* (p. **73**)

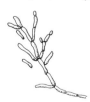

---

*Morphology alone cannot be relied upon for identification. Use procedure on
p. 218 and Tables 4.1–4.4 (pp. 64, 66, 76, and 79) for identification of genus and
species.

Yeastlike at 25–30°C and also at 35–37°C if growth occurs (*continued*)
**All rapid growers except *Ustilago* spp.**
**All WHITE, CREAM, or TAN except *Rhodotorula* and *Sporobolomyces* spp.**

Microscopic morphology on Cornmeal-Tween 80 agar (Dalmau plate)*

---

***Pseudohyphae with blastoconidia*** (*continued*)

*Candida zeylanoides* (p. **74**)                    *Saccharomyces* (p. **81**)

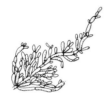

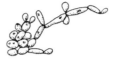

*Hansenula* (p. **82**)

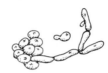

---

***Yeastlike cells only; usually no hyphae or pseudohyphae***

*Cryptococcus* (p. **75**)                    *Torulopsis* (p. **77**)

*Rhodotorula* (p. **78**)
(pink or coral pigment)

*Sporobolomyces* (p. **80**)
(pink or coral pigment)

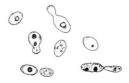

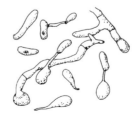

---

*Morphology alone cannot be relied upon for identification. Use procedure on p. 218 and Tables 4.1–4.4 (pp. 64, 66, 76, and 79) for identification of genus and species.

# MONOMORPHIC YEASTS AND YEASTLIKE ORGANISMS

Yeastlike at 25–30°C and also at 35–37°C if growth occurs (*continued*)
**All rapid growers except *Ustilago* spp.**
**All WHITE, CREAM, or TAN except *Rhodotorula* and *Sporobolomyces* spp.**

Microscopic morphology on Cornmeal-Tween 80 agar (Dalmau plate)*

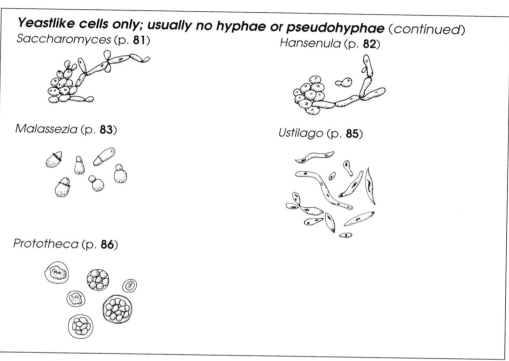

*Yeastlike cells only; usually no hyphae or pseudohyphae* (*continued*)
Saccharomyces (p. **81**)     Hansenula (p. **82**)

Malassezia (p. **83**)     Ustilago (p. **85**)

Prototheca (p. **86**)

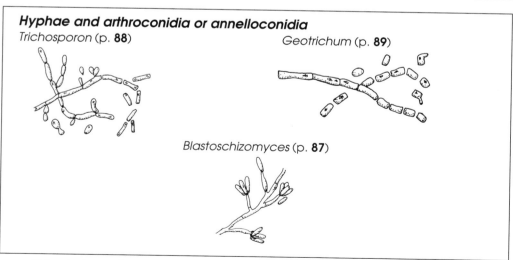

*Hyphae and arthroconidia or annelloconidia*
Trichosporon (p. **88**)     Geotrichum (p. **89**)

Blastoschizomyces (p. **87**)

*Morphology alone cannot be relied upon for identification. Use procedure on p. 218 and Tables 4.1–4.4 (pp. 64, 66, 76, and 79) for identification of genus and species.

## THERMALLY DIMORPHIC FUNGI

Filamentous when cultured at 25–30°C; yeastlike when cultured at 35–37°C*

| *Sporothrix schenckii* (p. 92) | *Histoplasma capsulatum* (p. 94) | *Blastomyces dermatitidis* (p. 96) | *Paracocci-dioides brasiliensis* (p. 98) | *Penicillium marneffei* (p. 100) |
|---|---|---|---|---|
| **25°C mold phase on Sabouraud dextrose agar** | | | | |
| MACROSCOPICALLY: | | | | |
| Wrinkled, leathery, some short aerial mycelium when old | Loose, cottony | Smooth, then prickly, then cottony | Heaped; short mycelium | Flat, velvety |
| White, then tan or black | White or brownish | White, then brownish | White, then brownish | Tan, then reddish-yellow and bluish green; red diffusing pigment |
| MICROSCOPICALLY: | | | | |
| Fine, branched, septate hyphae, ''flowerette'' conidial form | Branched, septate hyphae; microconidia; knobby macroconidia in 3–4 weeks | Branched, septate hyphae, single small conidia | Septate hyphae, chlamydo-conidia, few microconidia | Septate hyphae, metulae, phialides, chains of conidia |

**37°C yeast phase on brain heart infusion agar**
MACROSCOPICALLY: All cream or tan

| | | | | |
|---|---|---|---|---|
| MICROSCOPICALLY: | | | | |
| Round, oval, or ''cigar''-shaped | Small budding cells | Large, double-contoured cells budding on a broad base | Large, multiple budding cells, ''ship's wheel'' | Oval cells with central septum; no budding |

*See p. 220 for method of converting filamentous forms to yeast phase.

# THERMALLY MONOMORPHIC MOLDS

Filamentous when cultured at 25–30°C and also at 35–37°C if growth occurs
**SURFACE:** WHITE, CREAM, OR LIGHT GRAY*
**REVERSE:** NONPIGMENTED

---

## Having microconidia or macroconidia

Streptomyces** (p. **57**)

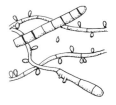

Microsporum vanbreuseghemii (p. **169**)

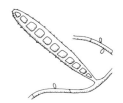

Trichophyton ajelloi (p. **182**)

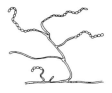

Trichophyton mentagrophytes (p. **171**)

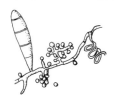

Trichophyton rubrum (p. **173**)

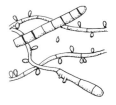

Trichophyton tonsurans (p. **174**)

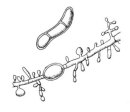

Trichophyton terrestre (p. **176**)

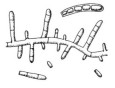

Fusarium (p. **201**)

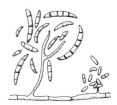

---

\* Also see p. 24, as several thermally dimorphic fungi may fit this description at 25–30°C.

\*\* *Streptomyces* is a filamentous bacterium.

**SURFACE:** WHITE, CREAM, OR LIGHT GRAY*
**REVERSE:** NONPIGMENTED (*continued*)

---

***Having microconidia or macroconidia*** (*continued*)

Acremonium (p. **200**)

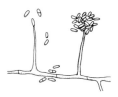

Verticillium (p. **199**)

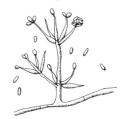

Beauveria (p. **198**)

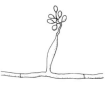

Pseudallescheria boydii (p. **132**)
(*Scedosporium apiospermum*)

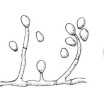

Chrysosporium (p. **203**)

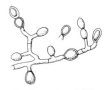

Emmonsia** (p. **188**)

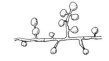

Sepedonium (p. **205**)

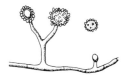

Graphium (p. **146**)

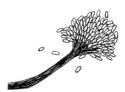

Stachybotrys (p. **145**)

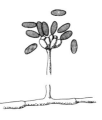

---

*Also see p. 24, as several thermally dimorphic fungi may fit this description at 25–30°C.
**Adiaspores form at ≥37°C.

**SURFACE:** WHITE, CREAM, OR LIGHT GRAY
**REVERSE:** NONPIGMENTED (*continued*)

## *Having sporangia or sporangiola*

Mucor (p. **107**)

Rhizopus (p. **108**)

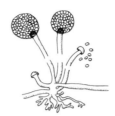

Rhizomucor (p. **110**)

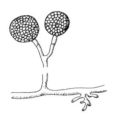

Absidia (p. **111**)

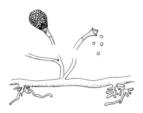

Apophysomyces (p. **112**)

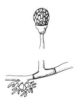

Saksenaea (p. **114**)

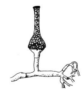

Cunninghamella (p. **116**)

Basidiobolus (p. **118**)

**SURFACE:** WHITE, CREAM, OR LIGHT GRAY*
**REVERSE:** NONPIGMENTED (*continued*)

---

***Having sporangia or sporangiola*** (*continued*)
*Conidiobolus* (p. **119**)

---

***Having arthroconidia***

*Geotrichum* (p. **89**)

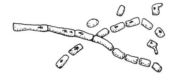

*Coccidioides* (p. **186**)

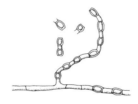

---

***Having only hyphae with chlamydoconidia***

*Microsporum ferrugineum* (p. **170**)

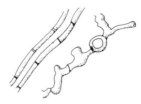

*Trichophyton schoenleini* (p. **178**)

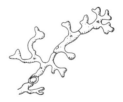

*Trichophyton verrucosum* (p. **179**)

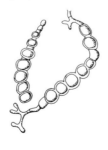

*Trichophyton violaceum* (p. **181**)

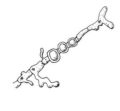

---

* Also see p. 24, as several thermally dimorphic fungi may fit this description at 25–30°C.

# THERMALLY MONOMORPHIC MOLDS

**SURFACE:** WHITE, CREAM, BEIGE, OR LIGHT GRAY
**REVERSE:** YELLOW, ORANGE, OR REDDISH

*Microsporum audouini* (p. **162**)

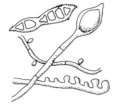

*Microsporum canis* var. *canis* (p. **163**)

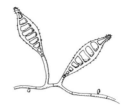

*Microsporum canis* var. *distortum* (p. **164**)

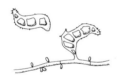

*Microsporum gypseum* (p. **166**)

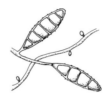

*Microsporum nanum* (p. **168**)

*Microsporum vanbreuseghemii* (p. **169**)

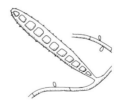

*Trichophyton mentagrophytes* (p. **171**)

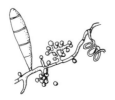

*Trichophyton rubrum* (p. **173**)

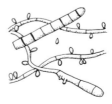

**SURFACE:** WHITE, CREAM, BEIGE, OR LIGHT GRAY
**REVERSE:** YELLOW, ORANGE, OR REDDISH (*continued*)

*Trichophyton tonsurans* (p. **174**)

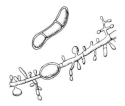

*Trichophyton terrestre* (p. **176**)

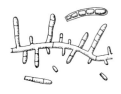

*Trichophyton verrucosum* (p. **179**)

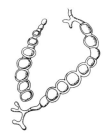

*Trichophyton schoenleini* (p. **178**)

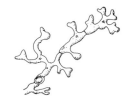

*Acremonium* (p. **200**)

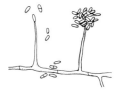

*Chaetomium* (p. **158**)

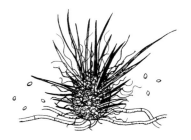

# THERMALLY MONOMORPHIC MOLDS

**SURFACE:** WHITE, CREAM, BEIGE, OR LIGHT GRAY
**REVERSE:** DEEP RED TO PURPLE

*Microsporum gypseum* (p. **166**)

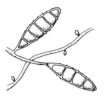

*Microsporum cookei* (p. **165**)

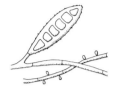

*Microsporum gallinae* (p. **167**)

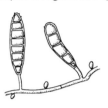

*Trichophyton ajelloi* (p. **182**)

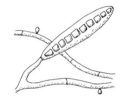

*Trichophyton rubrum* (p. **173**)

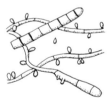

*Trichophyton megninii* (p. **175**)

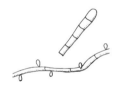

*Trichophyton mentagrophytes* (p. **171**)

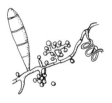

*Penicillium marneffei** (p. **100**)

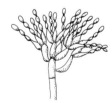

---

* *P. marneffei* is thermally dimorphic.

**SURFACE:** WHITE, CREAM, BEIGE, OR LIGHT GRAY
**REVERSE:** BROWNISH

*Madurella mycetomatis* (p. **140**)

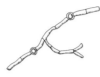

*Microsporum audouini* (p. **162**)

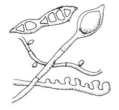

*Microsporum ferrugineum* (p. **170**)

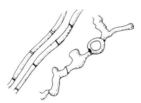

*Trichophyton schoenleini* (p. **178**)

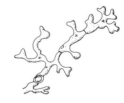

*Microsporum canis* (p. **163**)

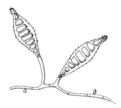

*Microsporum gypseum* (p. **166**)

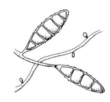

*Microsporum nanum* (p. **168**)

*Trichophyton mentagrophytes*
(p. **171**)

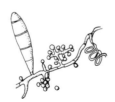

*Trichophyton rubrum* (p. **173**)

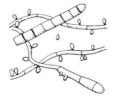

*Trichophyton tonsurans* (p. **174**)

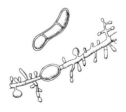

# THERMALLY MONOMORPHIC MOLDS

**SURFACE:** WHITE, CREAM, BEIGE, OR LIGHT GRAY
**REVERSE:** BROWNISH (*continued*)

Trichophyton terrestre (p. **176**)

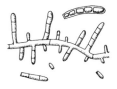

Scopulariopsis (p. **195**)

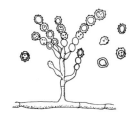

Chrysosporium (p. **203**)

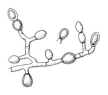

Emmonsia* (p. **188**)

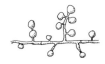

Sporotrichum (p. **204**)

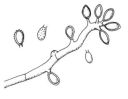

Cokeromyces (p. **115**)

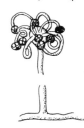

Chaetomium (p. **158**)

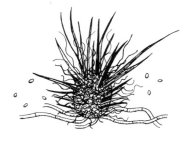

---

* Adiaspores form at ≥37°C.

**SURFACE:** WHITE, CREAM, BEIGE, OR LIGHT GRAY
**REVERSE:** BLACKISH

*Pseudallescheria boydii* (p. **132**)
   (*Scedosporium apiospermum*)

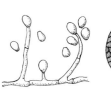

*Scedosporium prolificans* (p. **134**)

*Chaetomium* (p. **158**)

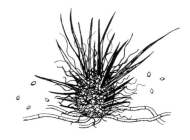

*Phoma* (p. **159**)

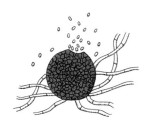

*Graphium* (p. **146**)

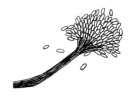

*Nigrospora* (p. **157**)

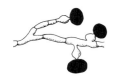

*Trichophyton ajelloi* (p. **182**)

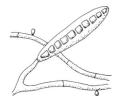

### Having small conidia

Aspergillus (p. **192**)

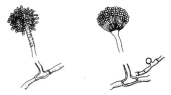

Trichophyton tonsurans (p. **174**)

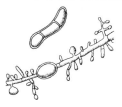

Cladosporium carrioni (p. **128**)

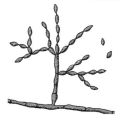

Cladosporium spp. (p. **130**)

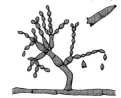

Paecilomyces (p. **194**)

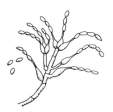

Scopulariopsis (p. **195**)

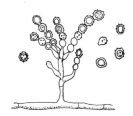

Verticillium (p. **199**)

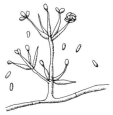

Pseudallescheria boydii (p. **132**)
(*Scedosporium apiospermum*)

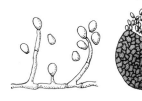

Emmonsia** (p. **188**)

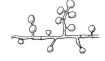

Chrysosporium (p. **203**)

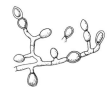

*Also see p. 24, as several thermally dimorphic fungi may fit this description at 25-30°C.
**Adiaspores form at ≥37°C.

**SURFACE:** TAN TO BROWN* (*continued*)

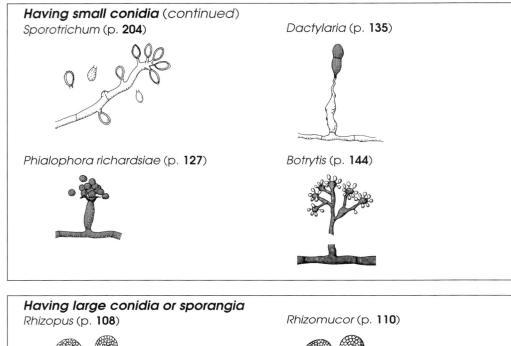

*Having small conidia* (*continued*)

Sporotrichum (p. **204**)

Dactylaria (p. **135**)

Phialophora richardsiae (p. **127**)

Botrytis (p. **144**)

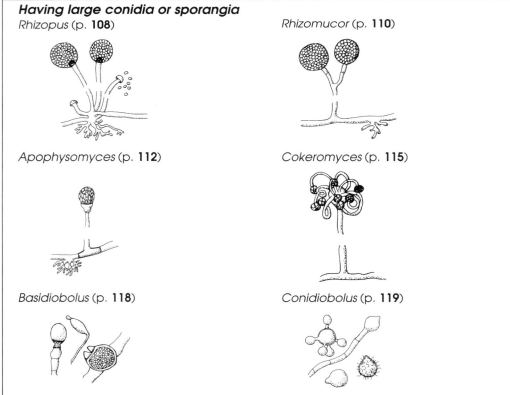

*Having large conidia or sporangia*

Rhizopus (p. **108**)

Rhizomucor (p. **110**)

Apophysomyces (p. **112**)

Cokeromyces (p. **115**)

Basidiobolus (p. **118**)

Conidiobolus (p. **119**)

*Also see p. 24, as several thermally dimorphic fungi may fit this description at 25-30°C.

**SURFACE:** TAN TO BROWN* (*continued*)

### Having large conidia or sporangia (*continued*)

Alternaria (p. **152**)

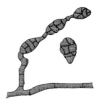

Stemphylium (p. **154**)

Ulocladium (p. **153**)

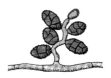

Epicoccum (p. **156**)

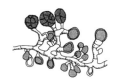

Curvularia (p. **147**)

Bipolaris (p. **148**)

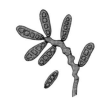

Microsporum gypseum (p. **166**)

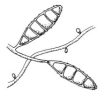

Microsporum cookei (p. **165**)

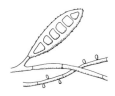

Microsporum nanum (p. **168**)

Microsporum vanbreuseghemii (p. **169**)

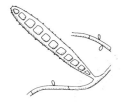

---

* Also see p. 24, as several thermally dimorphic fungi may fit this description at 25–30°C.

**SURFACE:** TAN TO BROWN* (*continued*)

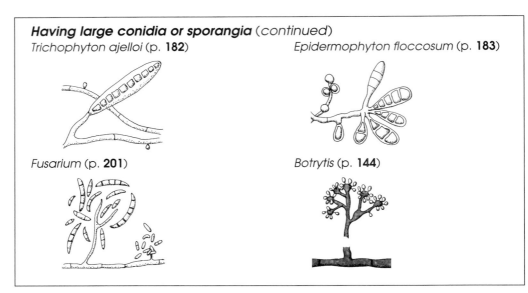

**Having large conidia or sporangia** (*continued*)

Trichophyton ajelloi (p. **182**)

Epidermophyton floccosum (p. **183**)

Fusarium (p. **201**)

Botrytis (p. **144**)

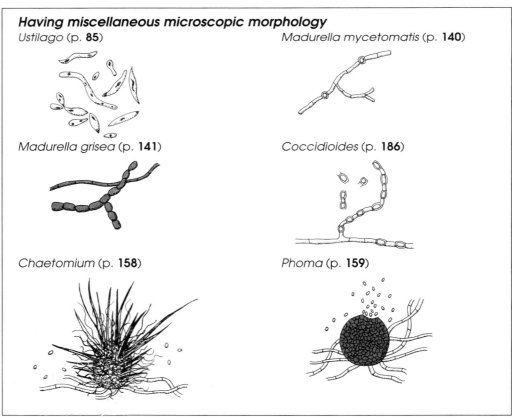

**Having miscellaneous microscopic morphology**

Ustilago (p. **85**)

Madurella mycetomatis (p. **140**)

Madurella grisea (p. **141**)

Coccidioides (p. **186**)

Chaetomium (p. **158**)

Phoma (p. **159**)

*Also see p. 24, as several thermally dimorphic fungi may fit this description at 25–30°C.

**SURFACE:** YELLOW TO ORANGE

Nocardia* (p. **55**)

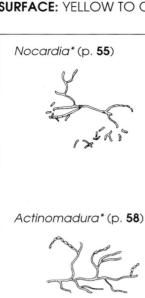

Streptomyces* (p. **57**)

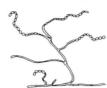

Actinomadura* (p. **58**)

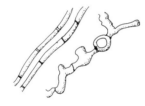

Nocardiopsis* (p. **59**)

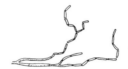

Microsporum ferrugineum (p. **170**)

Trichophyton tonsurans (p. **174**)

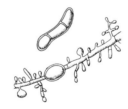

Trichophyton verrucosum (p. **179**)

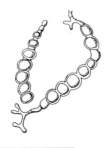

Trichophyton terrestre (p. **176**)

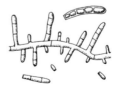

*These organisms are actinomycetes.

**SURFACE:** YELLOW TO ORANGE (*continued*)

*Trichophyton soudanense* (p. **177**)

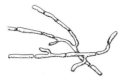

*Microsporum cookei* (p. **165**)

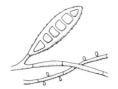

*Trichophyton ajelloi* (p. **182**)

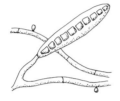

*Epidermophyton floccosum* (p. **183**)

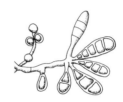

*Aspergillus* (p. **192**)

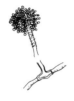

*Penicillium marneffei** (p. **100**)

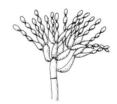

*Verticillium* (p. **199**)

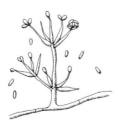

*Trichothecium* (p. **202**)

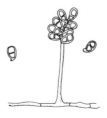

***P. marneffei* is thermally dimorphic.

**SURFACE:** YELLOW TO ORANGE (*continued*)

Chrysosporium (p. **203**)

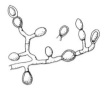

Sporotrichum (p. **204**)

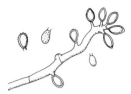

Sepedonium (p. **205**)

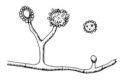

Monilia sitophila (p. **206**)

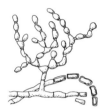

Epicoccum (p. **156**)

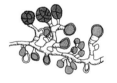

# THERMALLY MONOMORPHIC MOLDS

**SURFACE:** PINK TO VIOLET

Streptomyces* (p. **57**)
   (or Actinomadura, p. **58**)

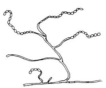

Microsporum cookei (p. **165**)
   (grape-red)

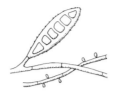

Microsporum gallinae (p. **167**)

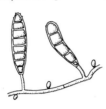

Microsporum vanbreuseghemii (p. **169**)

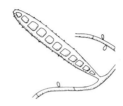

Trichophyton mentagrophytes (p. **171**)

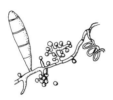

Trichophyton megninii (p. **175**)

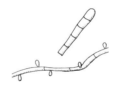

Trichophyton tonsurans (p. **174**)

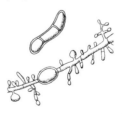

Trichophyton soudanense (p. **177**)

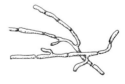

Trichophyton violaceum (p. **181**)

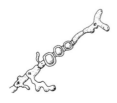

Aspergillus versicolor (p. **190**)

---

\* *Streptomyces* and *Actinomadura* are filamentous bacteria.

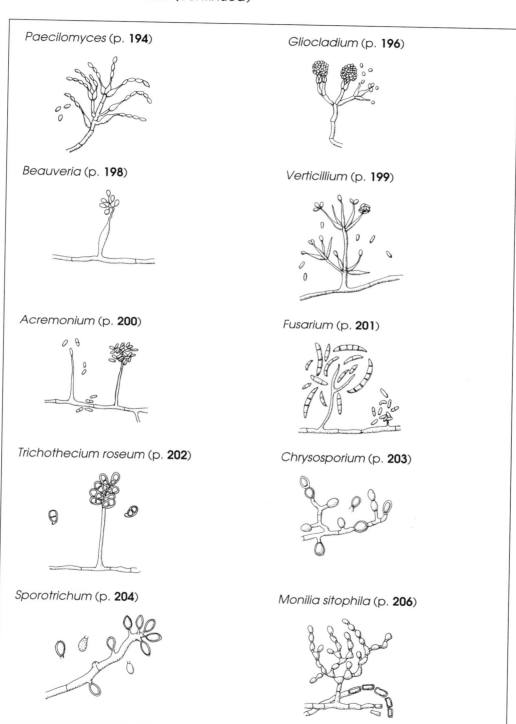

Paecilomyces (p. **194**)

Gliocladium (p. **196**)

Beauveria (p. **198**)

Verticillium (p. **199**)

Acremonium (p. **200**)

Fusarium (p. **201**)

Trichothecium roseum (p. **202**)

Chrysosporium (p. **203**)

Sporotrichum (p. **204**)

Monilia sitophila (p. **206**)

**SURFACE:** GREEN
**REVERSE:** LIGHT

*Aspergillus fumigatus, A. flavus, A. versicolor, A. nidulans, A. glaucus,* or *A. clavatus* (p. **192**)

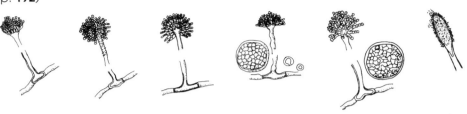

*Penicillium* (p. **193**)

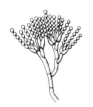

*Gliocladium* (p. **196**)

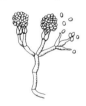

*Trichoderma* (p. **197**)

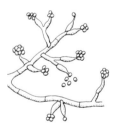

*Verticillium* (p. **199**)

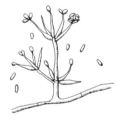

*Epidermophyton floccosum* (p. **183**)

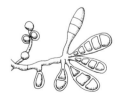

# THERMALLY MONOMORPHIC MOLDS

**SURFACE:** DARK GRAY OR BLACK
**REVERSE:** LIGHT

*Syncephalastrum* (p. **117**)

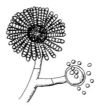

*Aspergillus niger* (p. **190**)

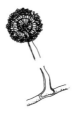

# THERMALLY MONOMORPHIC MOLDS

**SURFACE:** GREENISH, DARK GRAY, OR BLACK
**REVERSE:** DARK

## *Having small conidia**

*Fonsecaea pedrosoi* (p. **123**)

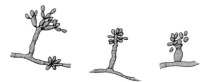

*Fonsecaea compacta* (p. **125**)

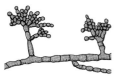

*Cladosporium* sp. (p. **130**)

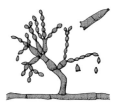

*Cladosporium carrionii* (p. **128**)

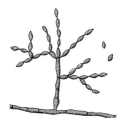

*Xylohypha bantiana* (p. **131**)

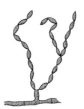

*Exophiala jeanselmi* (p. **136**)

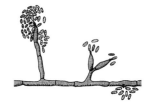

*Wangiella dermatitidis* (p. **137**)

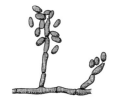

*Phaeoannellomyces werneckii* (p. **139**)

*Also see p. 92, as *Sporothrix schenckii* may fit this description at 25–30°C.

**SURFACE:** GREENISH, DARK GRAY, OR BLACK
**REVERSE:** DARK (*continued*)

### *Having small conidia** (*continued*)

Aureobasidium pullulans (p. **143**)

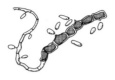

Phialophora verrucosa (p. **126**)

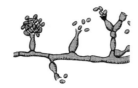

Phialophora richardsiae (p. **127**)

Scedosporium prolificans (p. **134**)

Pseudallescheria boydii (p. **132**)
(*Scedosporium apiospermum*)

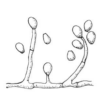

Botrytis (p. **144**)

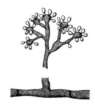

*Also see p. 92, as *Sporothrix schenckii* may fit this description at 25–30°C.

**SURFACE:** GREENISH, DARK GRAY, OR BLACK
**REVERSE:** DARK (*continued*)

### Having large conidia

Bipolaris (p. **148**)

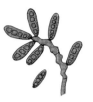

Curvularia (p. **147**)

Helminthosporium (p. **151**)

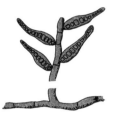

Dactylaria (p. **135**)

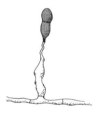

Stachybotrys (p. **145**)

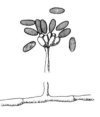

Alternaria (p. **152**)

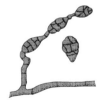

Stemphylium (p. **154**)

Ulocladium (p. **153**)

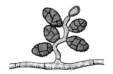

# THERMALLY MONOMORPHIC MOLDS

**SURFACE:** GREENISH, DARK GRAY, OR BLACK
**REVERSE:** DARK (*continued*)

---

### Having large conidia (*continued*)

Pithomyces (p. **155**)

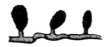

Epicoccum (p. **156**)

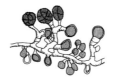

Nigrospora (p. **157**)

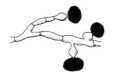

---

### Having only hyphae (with or without chlamydoconidia)

Madurella grisea (p. **141**)

Piedraia hortae (p. **142**)

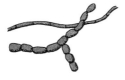

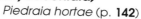
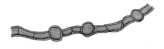

---

### Having large fruiting bodies

Chaetomium (p. **158**)

Phoma (p. **159**)

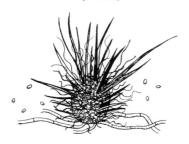

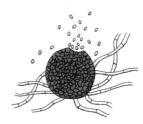

---

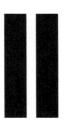

# Detailed Descriptions

# Filamentous Bacteria

# 3

The aerobic actinomycetes resemble fungi in that they form filaments that are well developed and branched (commonly referred to as hyphae). However, cell wall analysis, lack of a membrane-bound nucleus, lack of mitochondria, small size, and sensitivity to antibacterial agents define these organisms as bacteria rather than fungi.

The aerobic actinomycetes are gram positive and have filaments that are 1 µm or less in diameter. Some may be partially acid fast when stained by a modified Kinyoun method (p. 225). These organisms grow on mycology media without antibacterial additives and on routine mycobacteriology media. The colonies are usually glabrous and often become covered with a chalky or powdery coat. Microscopic morphology is best observed by slide culture on minimal medium such as cornmeal-Tween 80 agar or 2% plain agar prepared with tap water.

In addition to morphology and staining characteristics, a battery of biochemical tests can be used to differentiate the organisms in this group (see Table 3.1, p. 56). It is occasionally necessary to confirm an identification by cell wall analysis, which is accomplished with thin-layer chromatography or high-performance liquid chromatography. These procedures are available in some reference laboratories.

The most commonly encountered pathogenic aerobic actinomycetes belong to the genus *Nocardia*; they cause pulmonary, systemic, and cutaneous diseases, including mycetomas. Members of the other genera are etiologic agents of mycetoma; some *Streptomyces* spp. are considered nonpathogenic contaminants.

*For a complete review of the aerobic actinomycetes, see*
 *McNeil and Brown, 1994*
 *Murray et al., 1995, Manual of Clinical Microbiology, 6th ed., chapter 30*

**PATHOGENICITY:**  Causes nocardiosis, which symptomatically may be similar to tuberculosis or actinomycosis. Disease may begin as a pulmonary infection and later involve the central nervous system, kidneys, and other organs. Skin lesions or subcutaneous abscesses may be the only manifestation of infection; occasionally mycetomas develop in the extremities. On rare occasions, the eye has been infected. The organisms are ubiquitous in nature and may therefore be encountered as contaminants or colonizers.

**RATE OF GROWTH:**  Moderately rapid; mature in 7–9 days. Optimal growth is at 35–37°C. Grows on Sabouraud dextrose agar (SDA) without antibiotics and also on Lowenstein-Jensen and Middlebrook 7H11 media (frequently survives decontamination procedures used for isolation of acid-fast bacilli).

**COLONY MORPHOLOGY:**  Grows aerobically on SDA without antibiotics, forming raised, irregular, folded colonies varying from white to orange, depending on species. May be glabrous or develop a white chalky coating.

**MICROSCOPIC MORPHOLOGY:**  Delicate, branching, often beaded, intertwining filaments that fragment into bacillary and coccoid forms; best exhibited on slide culture using a minimal medium such as cornmeal-Tween 80 agar. They are gram positive and often, but not always, partially acid fast (use a modified Kinyoun method, p. 225). Young primary cultures are usually the most acid fast; acid fastness may be enhanced on Middlebrook 7H11 or by growing for 3–4 weeks in a proteinaceous medium such as litmus milk or bromocresol purple milk.

See Table 3.1 (p. 56) for differentiation of species.

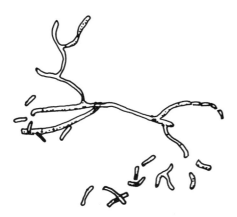

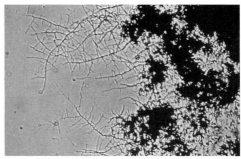

From ASM Teleconference of 9 August 1994, by Joseph Staneck, on Aerobic Actinomycetes: Nocardia and Related Organisms.

*For further information, see*
*Kwon-Chung and Bennett, 1992, pp. 582–588*
*McNeil and Brown, 1994*
*Rippon, 1988, pp. 53–68, 94–103*
*Wentworth, 1988, 271–302*

**TABLE 3.1** Differentiation of aerobic actinomycetes[a]

| Organism | Colony on Sabouraud dextrose agar | Fragmentation of hyphae[b] | Acid fast (partially) | Decomposition of:[c] | | | | | | Growth with lysozyme | Acid from: | | |
|---|---|---|---|---|---|---|---|---|---|---|---|---|---|
| | | | | Casein | Tyrosine | Xanthine | Urea | Gelatin | Starch | | Lactose | Xylose | Cellobiose |
| *Nocardia asteroides* | White to pink or orange; glabrous or powdery; wrinkled | + | + | 0 | 0 | 0 | + | 0[v] | 0[v] | + | 0 | 0 | 0 |
| *Nocardia brasiliensis* | White to pink or orange; glabrous or powdery; wrinkled | + | + | + | + | 0 | + | + | 0[v] | + | 0 | 0 | 0 |
| *Nocardia otitidiscaviarum*[d] | White to pink or orange; glabrous or powdery; wrinkled | + | + | 0 | 0[v] | + | + | 0 | 0[v] | + | 0 | 0 | 0 |
| *Nocardiopsis dassonvillei* | Yellowish, heaped, wrinkled; chalky or velvety | + | 0 | + | + | + | + | + | + | 0 | 0 | + | + |
| *Actinomadura madurae* | White to tan, pink, red, or orange; glabrous; wrinkled; hard; adherent; slow growing | 0 | 0 | + | +[v] | 0 | 0 | + | + | 0 | V | + | + |
| *Actinomadura pelletieri* | Bright red; heaped; glabrous | 0 | 0 | + | + | 0 | 0 | + | 0 | 0 | 0 | 0 | 0 |
| *Streptomyces somaliensis* | Cream to brown or black; slow growing; leathery; folded | 0 | 0 | + | + | 0 | 0 | + | V | 0 | 0 | 0 | 0 |
| *Streptomyces griseus* | White or grayish; glabrous, chalky, or velvety | 0 (spores often +) | 0 (spores often +) | + | + | + | + | + | + | 0 | + | + | + |
| *Streptomyces* spp. (*S. albus, S. lavendulae, S. rimosus*) | Variety of colors; glabrous, chalky, or velvety | 0 (spores often +) | 0 (spores often +) | + | + | +[v] | V | +[v] | +[v] | V | +[v] | V | V |

[a]Chromatographic analysis of cell walls or whole cells may be required (performed by reference laboratories). Abbreviations: +, positive; 0, negative; V, variable.

[b]Smears must be made with care to detect spontaneous fragmentation rather than that caused by trauma.

[c]Within 2 weeks at room temperature (25–30°C).

[d]Formerly *Nocardia caviae*.

**PATHOGENICITY:**   Some *Streptomyces* spp. are considered nonpathogenic contaminants. Other species, such as *S. somaliensis*, cause mycetomas and occasionally other types of infections. *S. griseus* is the most commonly isolated species, but it only occasionally appears to be an etiologic agent of infection.

**RATE OF GROWTH:**   Rapid or moderate; mature in 4–10 days. Optimum growth occurs at 30°C.

**COLONY MORPHOLOGY:**   Surface is slightly folded, hard, leathery; may develop a fine chalky or powdery aerial mycelium. Many strains have various pigments of gray, orange, rose, red, or occasionally green. Culture often produces the characteristic odor of freshly tilled soil.

**MICROSCOPIC MORPHOLOGY:**   Hyphae are long, thin (1 μm or less in diameter), and abundantly branching with filaments which may be straight, wavy, or spiraled. Small oblong conidia are produced at distinct points on the filament; this is best observed on slide culture. Some species do not form conidia readily.
   See Table 3.1 (p. 56) for differentiation of aerobic actinomycetes.

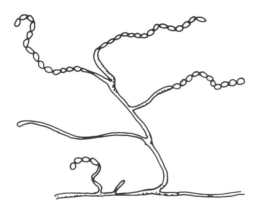

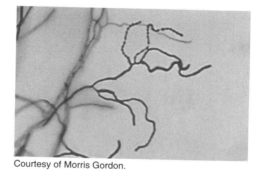

Courtesy of Morris Gordon.

*For further information, see*
   *Kwon-Chung and Bennett, 1992, pp. 584, 588*
   *McNeil and Brown, 1994*
   *Rippon, 1988, pp. 97–103*
   *Wentworth, 1988, pp. 271–302*
   *Wilson and Plunkett, 1970, pp. 153–155, 361–362*

## *Actinomadura* spp.

**PATHOGENICITY:**  A frequent cause of mycetoma; *A. madurae* is the second most common aerobic actinomycete encountered by the Centers for Disease Control and Prevention (*Nocardia asteroides* is the most common).

**RATE OF GROWTH:**  Usually rapid on Lowenstein-Jensen (L-J) medium, slower on Sabouraud dextrose agar. Optimum growth is at 35–37°C.

**COLONY MORPHOLOGY:**  Waxy, folded, membranous or mucoid. May be white, tan, pink, orange, or red. White aerial hyphae may develop after 2 weeks of incubation; best seen on L-J medium.

**MICROSCOPIC MORPHOLOGY:**  Narrow abundantly branched filaments (0.5 to 1 μm in diameter) that are gram positive, non-acid fast, and nonfragmenting. Short chains of round conidia may be produced from limited portions of the aerial hyphae; this is best observed on slide culture.

See Table 3.1 (p. 56) for differentiation of aerobic actinomycetes.

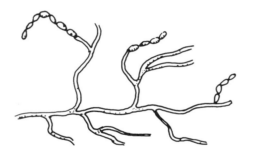 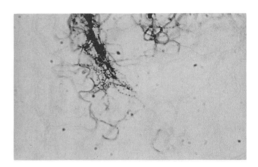

*For further information, see*
*Kwon-Chung and Bennett, 1992, pp. 582–585*
*McNeil and Brown, 1994*
*Rippon, 1988, pp. 97–102*
*Wentworth, 1988, pp. 289–299*

**PATHOGENICITY:**   Very occasional etiologic agent of mycetoma and other cutaneous infections.

**RATE OF GROWTH:**   Moderately rapid; mature in 4–10 days.

**COLONY MORPHOLOGY:**   Yellowish, heaped, irregularly wrinkled. Aerial hyphae develop to form a velvety coating.

**MICROSCOPIC MORPHOLOGY:**   Narrow filaments (1 μm or less in diameter) that are long, extensive, sometimes branched; they are gram positive and non-acid fast. The filaments fragment into chains of arthroconidia, giving a characteristic zigzag appearance. The total length of the aerial hyphae turns into conidial chains, in contrast to *Actinomadura* and *Streptomyces* spp., which produce conidial chains only at distinct parts of the hyphae.

See Table 3.1 (p. 56) for differentiation of aerobic actinomycetes.

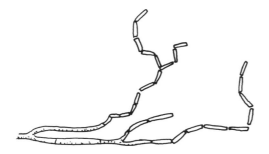
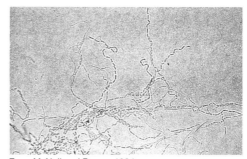

From McNeil and Brown, 1994.

*For further information, see*
  *Kwon-Chung and Bennett, 1992, pp. 582–588*
  *McNeil and Brown, 1994*
  *Rippon, 1988, pp. 98, 102*

# Yeasts and Yeastlike Organisms

# 4

In this Guide, the terms "yeast" and "yeastlike" refer to unicellular organisms that generally reproduce by budding. If the buds (blastoconidia) elongate and remain attached to the parent cell, they form chains known as pseudohyphae. Some of the organisms included here produce true septate hyphae while others form no hyphal elements of any sort. A few are capable of producing ascospores. Organisms that are actually molds or algae but that grow in a yeastlike manner are traditional members of this group.

Colonies are smooth and glabrous and may be moist or dry; they are usually white to cream colored, but some are tan, pinkish, or orangey.

The ability to produce pseudohyphae, true hyphae, and/or terminal chlamydospores and the shape and arrangement of blastoconidia are used along with other morphologic characteristics and biochemical tests to identify the yeasts to the genus and species level. A number of commercial systems are available for biochemical testing (see p. 218). Microscopic morphology is studied on agar such as cornmeal-Tween 80 agar by using the Dalmau method (p. 241), which ensures the decreased oxygen environment required for the production of structures used for identification.

Yeasts are the most common fungi isolated in the clinical laboratory. They are ubiquitous in our environment and also live as normal inhabitants in our bodies, so it is often difficult to determine the clinical significance of an isolate. Implication of the yeast as the etiologic agent of infection often requires repeated recovery from the site and direct microscopic demonstration of the yeast in infected tissue. The yeasts and yeastlike organisms are considered opportunistic pathogens, causing disease in patients (i) with a breakdown in the body's immune system; (ii) on prolonged treatment with antibiotics, corticosteroids, or cytotoxic drugs; (iii) with intravascular catheters; (iv) with diabetes mellitus; or (v) known to be intravenous drug abusers.

*For further information, see*
  *Murray et al., 1995, Manual of Clinical Microbiology, 6th ed., chapter 60*

**PATHOGENICITY:** Most common cause of candidiasis (candidosis), which is an acute, subacute, or chronic infection involving any part of the body. This organism may also be found as normal flora in the skin, mouth, vaginal mucous membranes, and stools.

**RATE OF GROWTH:** Rapid; mature in 3 days.

**COLONY MORPHOLOGY:** Cream colored, pasty, smooth.

**MICROSCOPIC MORPHOLOGY:** On cornmeal-Tween 80 agar (Dalmau plate, p. 241) at 25°C for 72 h, pseudohyphae (and some true hyphae) with clusters of round blastoconidia at the septa and large, thick-walled terminal chlamydospores. Chlamydospore formation is inhibited at 30–37°C. *C. albicans* gives a positive reaction to the germ-tube test (p. 219).

Blastoconidia of *Candida* spp. are approx 3–7 × 3–14 µm.

*C. stellatoidea* (usually considered a subspecies of *C. albicans*) is morphologically similar to *C. albicans* but differs mainly by not assimilating sucrose and not tolerating cycloheximide.

See Tables 4.1 (p. 64) and 4.2 (p. 66) for differentiation of yeastlike genera and characteristics of *Candida* species.

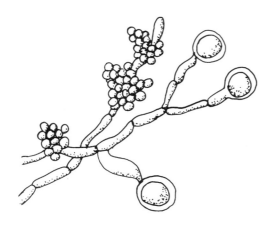
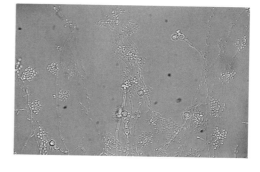

*For further information, see*
  *Kwon-Chung and Bennett, 1992, pp. 280–326*
  *Rippon, 1988, pp. 532–570*

**TABLE 4.1** Characteristics of the genera of clinically encountered yeasts and yeastlike organisms[a]

| Organism | On cornmeal-Tween 80 agar at 25°C | | | | | Asco-spores | Sporangia | Capsule | Urease | Growth: | | |
| | Pseudo-hyphae | True hyphae | Blastoconidia along hyphae | Arthro-conidia | Annello-conidia | | | | | With cycloheximide at 25°C | On SDA at 37°C | In Sabouraud broth |
|---|---|---|---|---|---|---|---|---|---|---|---|---|
| *Candida* | + | Few | + | 0 | 0 | 0 | 0 | 0 | $0^v$ | V | $+^v$ | Some species show surface growth |
| *Torulopsis* | 0 | 0 | | 0 | 0 | 0 | 0 | 0 | 0 | 0 | + | NSG |
| *Rhodotorula* | $0^R$ | 0 | | 0 | 0 | 0 | 0 | V | + | $0^v$ | $+^v$ | NSG |
| *Cryptococcus* | $0^R$ | 0 | | 0 | 0 | 0 | 0 | + | + | 0 | V | NSG |
| *Saccharomyces* | V | 0 | | 0 | 0 | + | 0 | 0 | 0 | 0 | + | NSG |
| *Hansenula* | $0^v$ | 0 | | 0 | 0 | + | 0 | 0 | 0 | 0 | V | NSG |
| *Malassezia* | $0^R$ | $0^R$ | | 0 | 0 | 0 | 0 | 0 | + | $+^{w,v}$ | $+^v$ | NSG |
| *Prototheca* | 0 | 0 | | 0 | 0 | 0 | + | $0^v$ | 0 | 0 | $+^v$ | Surface growth |
| *Geotrichum* | 0 | + | 0 | + | 0 | 0 | 0 | 0 | 0 | 0 | $0^w$ | Pellicle forms |
| *Trichosporon* | + | + | + | + | 0 | 0 | 0 | 0 | $+^v$ | $+^v$ | $+^v$ | Pellicle forms |
| *Blastoschizomyces* | + | + | + | $0^v$ | + | 0 | 0 | 0 | 0 | + | + | Pellicle forms |

[a]Abbreviations: SDA, Sabouraud dextrose agar; +, positive; 0, negative; V, species or strain variation; W, weak; R, rarely few rudimentary forms; NSG, no surface growth.

**PATHOGENICITY:** As is true of many species of *Candida* and other yeasts, *C. tropicalis* is known to cause infection, especially in immunocompromised, predisposed patients, as discussed on p. 62. It is also found without evidence of disease.

**RATE OF GROWTH:** Rapid; mature in 3 days.

**COLONY MORPHOLOGY:** Creamy with mycelial fringe.

**MICROSCOPIC MORPHOLOGY:** On cornmeal-Tween 80 agar at 25°C for 72 h, it forms blastoconidia singly or in very small groups all along graceful, long pseudohyphae. True hyphae may also be present. A few teardrop-shaped chlamydospores may rarely be produced.

An organism which closely resembles *C. tropicalis* has been isolated from clinical specimens and given the name *Candida paratropicalis* (Baker et al., 1981). It physiologically differs only slightly from the sucrose-negative form of *C. tropicalis* and is not considered to be a separate species by some mycologists.

See Tables 4.1 (p. 64) and 4.2 (p. 66) for differentiation of yeastlike genera and characteristics of *Candida* species.

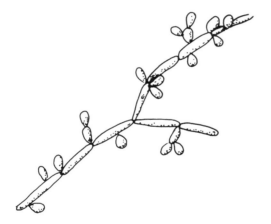 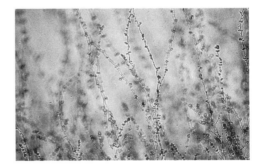

*For further information, see*
  *Kwon-Chung and Bennett, 1992, pp. 280–326*
  *Rippon, 1988, pp. 532–574*

**TABLE 4.2** Characteristics of *Candida* spp. most commonly encountered in the clinical laboratory[a]

| Organism | Microscopic morphology on cornmeal-Tween 80 agar at 25°C | Growth: | | | Germ tubes |
| | | In Sabouraud broth | With cycloheximide at 25°C | On SDA at 37°C | |
|---|---|---|---|---|---|
| C. albicans<br><br>C. stellatoidea | Pseudohyphae with terminal chlamydospores; clusters of blasto-conidia at septa | NSG | +<br><br>0 | + | + |
| C. tropicalis[c] | Blastoconidia anywhere along pseudohyphae | Narrow surface film with bubbles | 0$^v$ | + | 0 |
| C. parapsilosis | Blastoconidia along curved pseudohyphae; giant mycelial cells | NSG | 0 | + | 0 |
| C. lusitaniae | Short chains of elongate blastoconidia along curved pseudohyphae | NSG | 0 | + | 0 |
| C. guilliermondii | Fairly short, fine pseudohyphae; clusters of blastoconidia at septa | NSG | + | + | 0 |
| C. kefyr<br>(C. pseudotropicalis) | Elongated blastoconidia resembling "logs in a stream" along pseudohyphae | NSG | + | + | 0 |
| C. zeylanoides | Pseudohyphae give feather-like appearance at low power | Pellicle (delayed) | 0 | 0$^v$ | 0 |
| C. krusei | Pseudohyphae with cross-matchsticks or treelike blastoconidia | Wide surface film up sides of tube | 0 | + | 0 |
| C. lipolytica | Elongated blastoconidia in short chains along pseudohyphae | Pellicle (delayed) | | +$^v$ | 0 |

[a]Abbreviations: SDA, Sabouraud dextrose agar; +, positive; 0, negative; W, reaction may be weak; V, strain variation; NSG, no surface growth.

[b]Fermentation is demonstrated by the production of *gas* (acid does not indicate fermentation).

[c]C. paratropicalis differs from C. tropicalis by not fermenting sucrose and melezitose, not assimilating arabinose, and having variable ability to assimilate methyl-D-glucoside, sucrose, and melezitose.

| Urease (25°C) | Assimilation of: | | | | | | | | | | | | | Fermentation of:[b] | | | | | | |
|---|---|---|---|---|---|---|---|---|---|---|---|---|---|---|---|---|---|---|---|---|
| | Dextrose | Maltose | Sucrose | Lactose | Galactose | Melibiose | Cellobiose | Inositol | Xylose | Raffinose | Trehalose | Dulcitol | KNO$_3$ | Dextrose | Maltose | Sucrose | Lactose | Galactose | Trehalose | Cellobiose |
| 0 | + | + | +/0 | 0 | + | 0 | 0 | 0 | + | 0 | + | 0 | 0 | + | + | 0 | 0 | +$^w$/0 | +$^v$/0 | 0 |
| 0 | + | + | +$^v$ | 0 | + | 0 | +$^v$ | 0 | + | 0 | + | 0 | 0 | + | + | +$^v$ | 0 | +$^v$ | +$^v$ | 0 |
| 0 | + | + | + | 0 | + | 0 | 0 | 0 | + | 0 | + | 0 | 0 | + | 0 | 0 | 0 | V | 0 | 0 |
| 0 | + | + | + | 0 | + | 0 | + | 0 | + | 0 | + | 0 | 0 | + | 0 | V | 0 | + | V | + |
| 0 | + | + | + | 0 | + | + | + | 0 | + | + | + | + | 0 | + | 0 | +$^w$ | 0 | +$^w$ | +$^w$ | 0 |
| 0 | + | 0 | + | + | + | 0 | + | 0 | +$^v$ | + | 0 | 0 | 0 | + | 0 | + | + | + | 0 | 0 |
| 0 | + | 0 | 0 | 0 | 0$^v$ | 0 | 0$^v$ | 0 | 0 | 0 | + | 0 | 0 | 0$^w$ | 0 | 0 | 0 | 0 | 0$^v$ | 0 |
| +$^v$ | + | 0 | 0 | 0 | 0 | 0 | 0 | 0 | 0 | 0 | 0 | 0 | 0 | + | 0 | 0 | 0 | 0 | 0 | 0 |
| + | + | 0 | 0 | 0 | 0 | 0 | 0 | 0 | 0 | 0 | 0 | 0 | 0 | 0 | 0 | 0 | 0 | 0 | 0 | 0 |

**PATHOGENICITY:**  Has been known to cause infections in particularly susceptible individuals, as discussed on p. 62. It is a relatively frequent cause of candidal
endocarditis.

**RATE OF GROWTH:**  Rapid; mature in 3 days.

**COLONY MORPHOLOGY:**  Creamy, sometimes developing a lacy appearance.

**MICROSCOPIC MORPHOLOGY:**  On cornmeal-Tween 80 agar at 25°C for 72 h,
blastoconidia, singly or in small clusters, are seen along the pseudohyphae. Outstanding characteristics are the crooked or curved appearance of relatively short
pseudohyphae and the occasional presence of large hyphal elements called
"giant cells."

See Tables 4.1 (p. 64) and 4.2 (p. 66) for differentiation of yeastlike genera and
characteristics of *Candida* species.

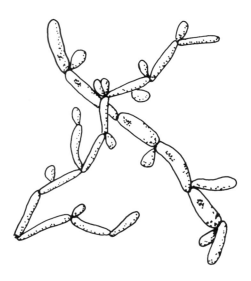
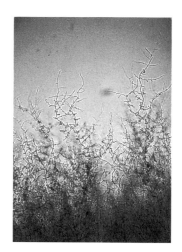

*For further information, see*
  *Kwon-Chung and Bennett, 1992, p. 319*

**PATHOGENICITY:** Encountered as an opportunistic pathogen in immunocompromised patients; development of resistance to amphotericin B has been frequently reported.

**RATE OF GROWTH:** Rapid; mature in 3 days.

**COLONY MORPHOLOGY:** Cream colored, smooth, glistening.

**MICROSCOPIC MORPHOLOGY:** On cornmeal-Tween 80 agar at 25°C for 72 h, pseudohyphae are slender, branched, and curved with short chains of elongate blastoconidia. Morphologically it resembles *C. tropicalis* and *C. parapsilosis* but differs by its ability to ferment cellobiose and assimilate rhamnose.

See Tables 4.1 (p. 64) and 4.2 (p. 66) for differentiation of yeastlike genera and characteristics of *Candida* species.

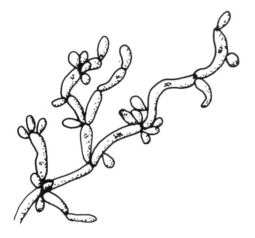 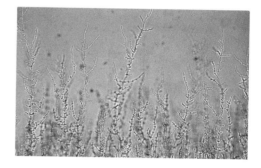

For further information, see
 Blinkhorn et al., 1989
 Kreger-van Rij, 1984, pp. 120–122
 Kwon-Chung and Bennett, 1992, pp. 318–319

**PATHOGENICITY:**  Known to cause infections in particularly susceptible individuals, as discussed on p. 62. It is resistant to fluconazole.

**RATE OF GROWTH:**  Rapid; mature in 3 days.

**COLONY MORPHOLOGY:**  Flat, dry, dull, developing a mycelial fringe. Cream colored.

**MICROSCOPIC MORPHOLOGY:**  On cornmeal-Tween 80 agar at 25° C for 72 h, it forms pseudohyphae with elongate blastoconidia forming a cross-matchsticks or treelike appearance.

The elongate blastoconidia of *C. krusei* may be confused with the annellides of *Blastoschizomyces capitatus*. *C. krusei* is sensitive to cycloheximide, ferments dextrose, and does not assimilate galactose. *B. capitatus* produces the opposite reactions.

See Tables 4.1 (p. 64) and 4.2 (p. 66) for differentiation of yeastlike genera and characteristics of *Candida* species.

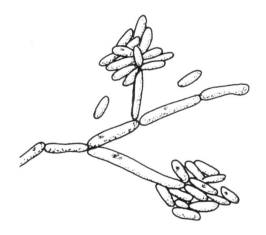
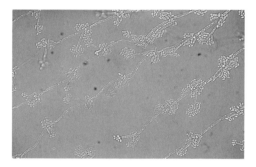

*For further information, see*
*Kreger-van Rij, 1984, pp. 726–728*
*Kwon-Chung and Bennett, 1992, pp. 316–318*

## Candida kefyr (C. pseudotropicalis)

**PATHOGENICITY:**  Usually considered nonpathogenic but sometimes causes infection in particularly susceptible individuals, as discussed on p. 62.

**RATE OF GROWTH:**  Rapid; mature in 3 days.

**COLONY MORPHOLOGY:**  Creamy, smooth.

**MICROSCOPIC MORPHOLOGY:**  On cornmeal-Tween 80 agar at 25°C for 72 h, it forms pseudohyphae with elongate blastoconidia that characteristically line up in parallel, giving the appearance of "logs in a stream."
   See Tables 4.1 (p. 64) and 4.2 (p. 66) for differentiation of yeastlike genera and characteristics of *Candida* species.

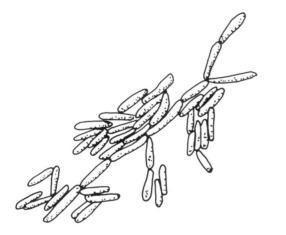 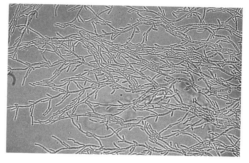

For further information, see
   Kwon-Chung and Bennett, 1992, pp. 316–317

**PATHOGENICITY:**  Usually considered nonpathogenic, but has been known to cause infection in particularly susceptible individuals, as described on p. 62.

**RATE OF GROWTH:**  Rapid; mature in 3 days.

**COLONY MORPHOLOGY:**  Flat, glossy, smooth edged, and usually cream colored, but may become pinkish with age.

**MICROSCOPIC MORPHOLOGY:**  On cornmeal-Tween 80 agar at 25°C for 72 h, it forms small yeast cells and relatively few, short pseudohyphae, often having small clusters of blastoconidia at the septa.

See Tables 4.1 (p. 64) and 4.2 (p. 66) for differentiation of yeastlike genera and characteristics of *Candida* species.

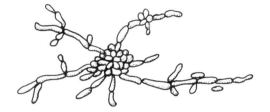
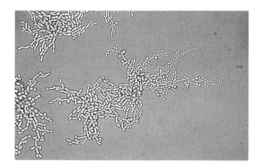

*For further information, see*
  *Kwon-Chung and Bennett, 1992, p. 315*

**PATHOGENICITY:**   An emerging opportunistic pathogen; may cause disease in the immunocompromised patient, as discussed on p. 62.

**RATE OF GROWTH:**   Rapid; mature in 6 days.

**COLONY MORPHOLOGY:**   Creamy, smooth, may be delicately wrinkled.

**MICROSCOPIC MORPHOLOGY:**   On cornmeal-Tween 80 agar at 25°C for 72 h, pseudohyphae and septate true hyphae bearing elongate blastoconidia in short chains form and produce a stark, branching appearance. Arthroconidia may be present.

   See Tables 4.1 (p. 64) and 4.2 (p. 66) for differentiation of yeastlike genera and characteristics of *Candida* species.

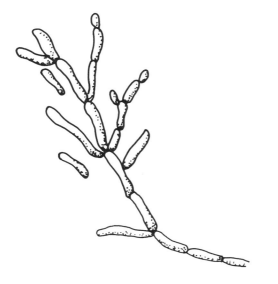 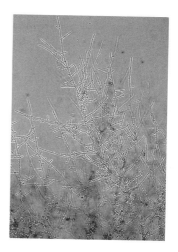

*For further information, see*
 *Kreger-van Rij, 1984, pp. 406–408*

**PATHOGENICITY:**   Rarely reported as cause of fungemia, arthritis, and skin and nail infections.

**RATE OF GROWTH:**   Rapid; mature in 3 days at 25–30°C; variable growth at 35–37°C.

**COLONY MORPHOLOGY:**   Smooth, dull, cream colored to yellowish.

**MICROSCOPIC MORPHOLOGY:**   On cornmeal-Tween 80 agar at 25°C for 72 h, pseudohyphae consist of cells that are frequently curved and bear oval or elongate blastoconidia singly and in small clusters and short chains. More blastoconidia are formed at the beginning of the pseudohyphae than at the distal end, creating a feather-like appearance at low power.

See Table 4.1 (p. 64) for differentiation of yeastlike genera and Table 4.2 (p. 66) for characteristics of *Candida* species.

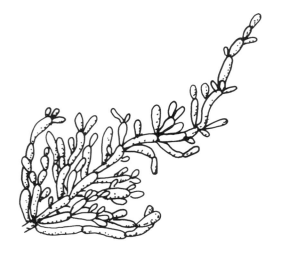
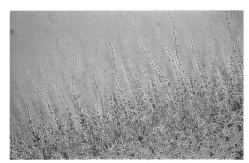

*For further information, see*
  *Kreger-van Rij, 1984, pp. 839–841*
  *Levenson et al., 1991*

**PATHOGENICITY:** Causes cryptococcosis, a subacute or chronic infection most frequently involving the tissue of the central nervous system but occasionally producing lesions in the skin, bones, lungs, or other internal organs. Cryptococcal meningitis is extremely common in AIDS patients. The other species of this genus are commonly considered nonpathogenic but may occasionally cause disease in severely immunosuppressed patients.

**RATE OF GROWTH:** Rapid; mature in 3 days.

**COLONY MORPHOLOGY:** Colonies are flat or slightly heaped, shiny, moist, and often mucoid, with smooth edges. Color is cream at first, later becoming tannish. Usually grows equally well at 25 and 37°C, whereas some of the other species of the genus will not grow well, if at all, at 37°C.

**MICROSCOPIC MORPHOLOGY:** On cornmeal-Tween 80 agar at 25°C for 72 h, cells (4–8 μm in diameter) are round, dark walled, and budding. Usually no hyphae are seen. Capsules are sometimes distinguishable on cornmeal-Tween 80 or on the germ tube test upon addition of India ink (p. 213). Production of capsular material may be increased by growth in 1% peptone solution. Some strains of *C. neoformans*, as well as other cryptococci, may not produce discernible capsules in vitro.

See Tables 4.1 (p. 64) and 4.3 (p. 76) for identification of genus and species. *C. neoformans* can be rapidly differentiated from other species of *Cryptococcus* by the caffeic acid test (p. 219).

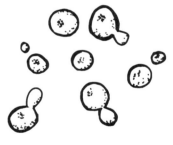
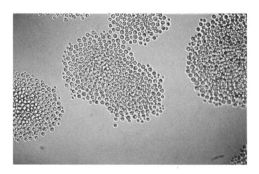

*For further information, see*
  *Kwon-Chung and Bennett, 1992, pp. 397–446*
  *McGinnis, 1980, pp. 389–392*
  *Rippon, 1988, pp. 582–609*

**TABLE 4.3** Characteristics of *Cryptococcus* spp.[a]

| Organism | Color on birdseed agar[b] | Growth at 37°C on SDA | Growth with cycloheximide at 25°C | Pseudo-hyphae (short) | Urease (25°C, 4 days) | Assimilation of: | | | | | | | | | | | | | Fermentation |
| --- | --- | --- | --- | --- | --- | --- | --- | --- | --- | --- | --- | --- | --- | --- | --- | --- | --- | --- | --- |
| | | | | | | Dextrose | Maltose | Sucrose | Lactose | Galactose | Melibiose | Cellobiose | Inositol | Xylose | Raffinose | Trehalose | Dulcitol | KNO$_3$ | |
| *C. neoformans* | Brown | + | 0 | 0[R] | + | + | + | + | 0 | + | 0 | +[v] | + | + | +[v] | + | + | 0 | |
| *C. uniguttulatus* | White | 0 | 0 | 0 | + | + | + | + | 0 | 0[v] | 0 | 0[v] | + | + | +[v] | +[v] | 0 | 0 | |
| *C. albidus var. albidus* | White | 0[v] | 0 | +[v] | + | + | + | + | +[v] | 0[v] | 0[v] | +[v] | + | + | +[w] | +[v] | +[v] | + | All species of *Cryptococcus* lack fermentative ability |
| *C. albidus var. diffluens* | White | +[v] | 0 | 0[v] | + | + | + | + | 0 | 0[v] | +[v] | +[v] | + | + | +[w] | +[v] | +[v] | + | |
| *C. laurentii* | White or greenish | + | 0[v] | 0 | + | + | + | + | + | + | +[v] | + | + | + | +[v] | +[v] | + | 0 | |
| *C. luteolus* | White | 0 | 0 | 0 | + | + | + | + | 0[v] | + | + | + | + | + | + | + | +[v] | 0 | |
| *C. terreus* | White | + | 0 | 0[v] | + | + | +[v] | 0[v] | 0[v] | +[v] | 0 | + | + | + | 0 | +[v] | +[v] | + | |
| *C. gastricus* | White | 0 | 0 | 0 | + | + | + | 0[v] | 0[v] | + | 0 | + | + | + | 0 | 0 | 0 | 0 | |

[a]Abbreviations: SDA, Sabouraud dextrose agar; +, positive; 0, negative; V, strain variation; R, occur rarely; W, reaction may be weak.
[b]The caffeic acid disk test (p. 219) is a rapid and sensitive alternative to birdseed agar.

**PATHOGENICITY:** Causes infections occurring usually in the bloodstream or urinary tract and sometimes in the lungs and other sites. The organism is also found in healthy individuals and appears to cause infection only in particularly susceptible persons, as discussed on p. 62.

**RATE OF GROWTH:** Rapid; mature in 3 days.

**COLONY MORPHOLOGY:** Small yeastlike colonies, pasty, smooth, white to cream.

**MICROSCOPIC MORPHOLOGY:** On cornmeal-Tween 80 agar at 25°C for 72 h, only small (2–3 × 4–5 μm), oval, single terminal budding, nonencapsulated yeast cells are seen. No pseudohyphae are formed.

See Tables 4.1 (p. 64) and 4.4 (p. 79) for differentiation of yeastlike fungi.

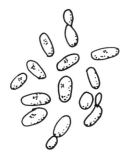
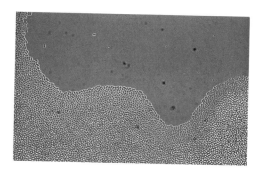

*For further information, see*
  *Kwon-Chung and Bennett, 1992, pp. 309–310, 314*
  *McGinnis, 1980, p. 398*
  *Rippon, 1988, p. 571*

**PATHOGENICITY:** Commonly known as a contaminant. Its presence in the terminal stages of debilitating diseases such as carcinoma and bacterial endocarditis may indicate an ability to colonize and infect particularly susceptible individuals.

**RATE OF GROWTH:** Rapid; mature in 4 days.

**COLONY MORPHOLOGY:** Usually pink to coral, but can also be orange, red, or yellow. Colony is yeastlike, soft, smooth, moist, and sometimes mucoid.

**MICROSCOPIC MORPHOLOGY:** On cornmeal-Tween 80 agar at 25°C for 72 h, budding cells that are round or oval and occasionally a few rudimentary pseudohyphae are seen. A faint capsule is sometimes formed. Cells measure 2–5.5 × 2.5–14 μm.
See Tables 4.1 (p. 64) and 4.4 (p. 79) for differentiation of yeastlike fungi.

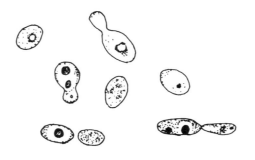 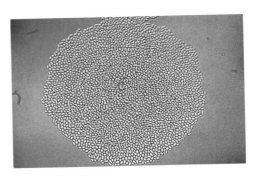

*For further information, see*
   *Kwon-Chung and Bennett,1992, pp. 770–773*
   *Rippon, 1988, pp. 610–611*

**TABLE 4.4**  Characteristics of yeasts and yeastlike organisms other than *Candida* spp. and *Cryptococcus* spp.[a]

| Organism | Microscopic morphology on cornmeal-Tween 80 agar at 25°C | Growth on SDA at 37°C | Asco-spores | Urease (25°C, 4 days) | Assimilation of: | | | | | | | | | | | | | Fermentation of: | | | | | | |
|---|---|---|---|---|---|---|---|---|---|---|---|---|---|---|---|---|---|---|---|---|---|---|---|---|
| | | | | | Dextrose | Maltose | Sucrose | Lactose | Galactose | Melibiose | Cellobiose | Inositol | Xylose | Raffinose | Trehalose | Dulcitol | KNO₃ | Dextrose | Maltose | Sucrose | Lactose | Galactose | Trehalose | Cellobiose |
| *Saccharomyces cerevisiae* | Occasional short pseudohyphae | + | + | 0 | + | +v | + | 0 | +v | 0 | 0 | 0 | 0 | + | +v | 0 | 0 | + | + | + | 0 | +v | +v | 0 |
| *Hansenula anomala* | May form pseudohyphae | V | + | 0 | + | + | + | 0 | +v | 0 | + | 0 | +v | +v | + | 0 | + | + | +v | + | 0 | +v | +v | V |
| *Geotrichum candidum* | True hyphae, arthroconidia, no blastoconidia | 0 | 0 | 0 | + | 0 | 0 | 0 | + | 0 | 0 | 0 | + | 0 | 0 | 0 | 0 | 0 | 0 | 0 | 0 | 0 | 0 | 0 |
| *Blastoschizomyces capitatus*[b] | Pseudohyphae and true hyphae, annelloconidia, few arthroconidia | + | 0 | 0 | + | 0 | 0 | 0 | + | 0 | 0 | 0 | 0 | 0 | 0 | 0 | 0 | 0 | 0 | 0 | 0 | 0 | 0 | 0 |
| *Trichosporon beigelii* | Pseudohyphae and true hyphae, arthroconidia, blastoconidia | +v | 0 | + | + | +v | +v | + | +v | +v | +v | +v | +v | +v | +v | +v | 0 | 0 | 0 | 0 | 0 | 0 | 0 | 0 |
| *Trichosporon pullulans* | Pseudohyphae and true hyphae, arthroconidia, blastoconidia | 0 | 0 | + | + | + | + | + | + | + | + | + | + | + | + | 0 | + | 0 | 0 | 0 | 0 | 0 | 0 | 0 |
| *Torulopsis glabrata* | No pseudohyphae, cells small, terminal budding | + | 0 | 0 | + | 0 | 0 | 0 | 0 | 0 | 0 | 0 | 0 | 0 | + | 0 | 0 | + | 0 | 0 | 0 | 0 | 0 | 0 |
| *Torulopsis* sp. | | 0v | 0 | 0 | + | 0v | +v | 0v | 0v | 0v | 0 | 0 | +v | + | + | 0v | 0v | +v | 0v | 0 | 0 | +v | 0 | 0 |
| *Rhodotorula rubra* | Usually no pseudohyphae | +v | 0 | + | + | + | + | 0 | +v | +v | +v | +v | + | + | + | 0v | 0v | 0 | 0 | 0 | 0 | 0v | 0 | 0 |
| *Rhodotorula glutinis* | | 0v | 0 | + | + | + | + | 0 | +v | +v | +v | + | +v | +v | + | 0 | 0 | 0 | 0 | 0 | 0 | 0 | 0 | 0 |
| *Sporobolomyces salmonicolor* | Ballistoconidia, various amounts of true and pseudohyphae | 0v | 0 | + | + | V | + | 0 | V | 0v | 0 | + | V | + | + | 0 | + | 0 | 0 | 0 | 0 | 0 | 0 | 0 |
| *Malassezia pachydermatis* | Usually no hyphae | + | 0 | + | + | 0 | 0 | 0 | 0 | 0 | 0 | 0 | 0 | 0 | 0 | 0 | + | Not done | | | | | | |
| *Prototheca wickerhamii* | Sporangia, no hyphae | + | 0 | 0 | + | 0 | 0 | +v | 0 | 0 | 0 | 0 | 0 | 0 | 0 | 0 | 0 | | | | | | | |
| *Prototheca zopfii* | | + | 0 | 0 | + | 0 | 0 | 0v | 0 | 0 | 0 | 0 | 0 | + | 0 | 0 | 0 | | | | | | | |
| *Prototheca stagnora* | | 0 | 0 | 0 | + | V | 0 | + | 0 | 0 | 0 | 0 | 0 | 0 | 0 | 0 | 0 | | | | | | | |

[a]Abbreviations: SDA, Sabouraud dextrose agar; +, positive; 0, negative; V, strain variation.
[b]Annelloconidia forming clusters at the ends of hyphae of *B. capitatus* may resemble the elongated blastoconidia of *Candida krusei*.

**PATHOGENICITY:**   Most commonly isolated from environmental sources. Very rarely reported as the cause of infection in immunocompromised patients.

**RATE OF GROWTH:**   Rapid, mature in 5 days. Best growth is at 25–30°C; may not grow well at 35–37°C.

**COLONY MORPHOLOGY:**   Smooth to slightly rough; characteristic salmon pink/coral color resembles that of *Rhodotorula* spp. (p. 78).

**MICROSCOPIC MORPHOLOGY:**   On cornmeal-Tween 80 agar at 25°C, oval to elongate yeastlike cells (2–12 × 3–35 µm) are seen; pseudohyphae and true hyphae may be absent or abundant. Kidney-shaped ballistoconidia (3–5 × 5–10 µm) are produced on denticles and are forcibly discharged, forming satellite colonies. Ballistoconidia can be best demonstrated by taping an inoculated cornmeal agar plate face to face to an uninoculated cornmeal plate. After extended incubation at 25°C, with the inoculated plate on top, the ballistoconidia that are shot off the inoculated plate will form a mirror image of colonies on the other plate.

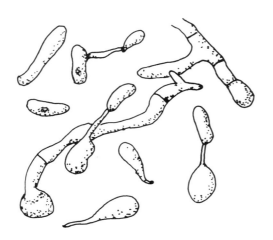 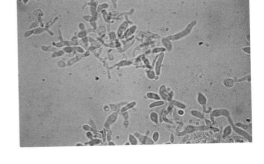

*For further information, see*
  *Kreger-van Rij, 1984, pp. 538–540, 911–920*
  *McGinnis, 1980, pp. 397–398*

**PATHOGENICITY:**   Usually considered nonpathogenic, but has been implicated in various infections in predisposed individuals.

**RATE OF GROWTH:**   Rapid; mature in 3 days.

**COLONY MORPHOLOGY:**   Smooth colonies, moist, white to cream colored.

**MICROSCOPIC MORPHOLOGY:**   On cornmeal-Tween 80 agar at 25°C for 72 h, yeast cells of various shapes with multilateral budding are seen. A few very short pseudohyphae may form. Cells measure approximately 3–9 × 5–20 μm.

   *Note*: Characteristic ascospores (1–4 per ascus) are best demonstrated when the organism is grown on a special medium, such as V-8 medium, acetate ascospore agar, or Gorodkowa medium (p. 234), and stained with ascospore stain (p. 227) or Kinyoun stain (p. 226). In addition, ascospores are gram negative, while vegetative cells are gram positive.

   See Tables 4.1 (p. 64) and 4.4 (p. 79) for differentiation of yeasts and yeastlike organisms.

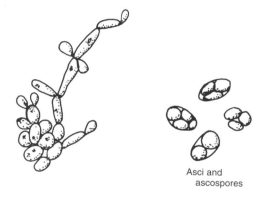

Asci and
ascospores

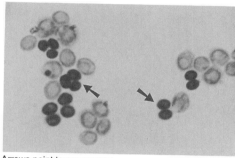

Arrows point to ascospores.

*For further information, see*
  *Kwon-Chung and Bennett, 1992, pp. 772–773*
  *McGinnis, 1980, p. 379*

## *Hansenula* spp.

**PATHOGENICITY:** Commonly considered a saprophyte; occasionally causes infection in predisposed patients.

**RATE OF GROWTH:** Rapid; mature in 3 days.

**COLONY MORPHOLOGY:** Smooth, moist, cream colored.

**MICROSCOPIC MORPHOLOGY:** On cornmeal-Tween 80 agar at 25°C for 72 h, budding yeast cells are seen (2–4 × 2–6 µm). Pseudohyphae form in some species. When cultured on ascospore medium (p. 234) and stained with Kinyoun (p. 226) or ascospore stain (p. 227), 1–4 ascospores per ascus are seen. There is a brim that turns downward around each ascospore, giving the impression of a helmet or hat.

See Tables 4.1 (p. 64) and 4.4 (p. 79) for identification.

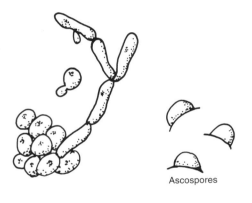

Ascospores

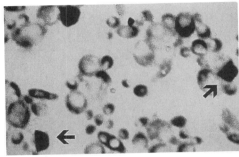

Arrows point to ascospores.

For further information, see
Kreger-van Rij, 1984, pp. 165–213
Kwon-Chung and Bennett, 1992, pp. 778–779
McGinnis, 1980, p. 377

**PATHOGENICITY:** Etiologic agent of pityriasis (tinea) versicolor, a superficial infection characterized by pale or dark patches of skin; medical attention is usually sought for cosmetic reasons. Folliculitis, resembling acne, occasionally occurs. Catheter-associated sepsis due to this organism is commonly seen in neonates and adults receiving prolonged intravenous lipids; pneumonia may develop in these patients. Rarely, the organism has been reported to cause peritonitis, septic arthritis, mastitis, sinusitis, and obstruction of the tear duct. *M. furfur* is part of the normal skin flora in over 90% of adults.

**RATE OF GROWTH:** Rapid; mature in 5 days at 30–37°C. Grows poorly at 25°C. The organism requires long-chain fatty acids for growth; solid medium overlaid with a thin film of olive oil is the most common method used.* Blood for culture must be taken through the lipid infusion catheter for best recovery of the organism; lysis-centrifugation (Isolator tubes, Wampole Laboratories) is advised as a result of many comparative studies.

**COLONY MORPHOLOGY:** Smooth, cream to yellowish brown; often becomes dry, dull, and lightly wrinkled with age.

**MICROSCOPIC MORPHOLOGY:** Yeastlike cells (1.5–4.5 × 2.0–6.5 μm) are actually phialides with small collarettes; the collarettes are very difficult to discern with a routine light microscope. The cells of this genus are unique in being round at one end and bluntly cut off at the other, where bud-like structures form singly on a broad base. There is no constriction at the point of budding. Hyphal elements are usually absent, but sparse rudimentary forms may occasionally develop.

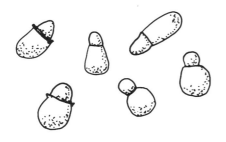
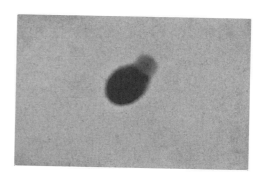

For further information, see
  Kwon-Chung and Bennett, 1992, pp.170–182
  Marcon and Powell, 1992

---

*M. furfur* can have its lipid requirement supplied by oleic acid or Tween 80; *M. sympodialis* cannot. This serves to distinguish *M. furfur* from the seldom encountered *M. sympodialis*.

**PATHOGENICITY:** More often found in lower animals than in humans; it has been associated with inflammation of ears of dogs. Occasionally reported to cause human infection, particularly in premature neonates receiving intravenous lipid emulsions.

**RATE OF GROWTH:** Rapid; mature in 5 days. Best growth is at 35–37°C; weak growth is seen at 25°C.

**COLONY MORPHOLOGY:** Creamy, dull, smooth; at first it is cream colored, becoming buff to orange-beige with age. Addition of fatty acids to the medium is NOT required for growth.

**MICROSCOPIC MORPHOLOGY:** On cornmeal-Tween 80 agar at 25°C for 72 h, cells are round to oval (2.5–5.5 $\times$ 3.0–6.5 µm); conidia are produced on a broad base at one pole, which develops a collarette. Pseudohyphae and true hyphae are usually absent, occasionally sparsely present. Biochemical yeast identification systems may misidentify this organism as *Candida lipolytica*; examination of microscopic morphology is essential.

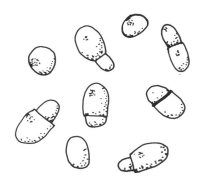

*For further information, see*
  *Kwon-Chung and Bennett, 1992, pp. 170–182*
  *Marcon and Powell, 1992*

**PATHOGENICITY:**   Parasitic on seeds and flowers of many cereals and grasses. May cause contamination in cultures. It has seldomly been implicated in human disease but may be inhaled and subsequently isolated from sputum specimens.

**RATE OF GROWTH:**   Slow; mature within 20 days.

**COLONY MORPHOLOGY:**   At first white, moist, pasty, and yeastlike; later it becomes tan to brown, wrinkled, raised, membranous, or velvety. Reverse is light in color.

**MICROSCOPIC MORPHOLOGY:**   Elongate, irregular, spindle-shaped or bean-pod-shaped yeastlike cells. Short hyphae with clamp connections are sometimes observed.

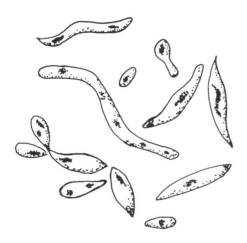

Courtesy of Michael McGinnis.

*For further information, see*
  *McGinnis, 1980, p. 386*
  *Wilson and Plunkett, 1970, p. 385*

## *Prototheca* spp.

(Actually an achlorophyllous alga; included in this guide because it causes mycosis-like infections and is often mistaken for a yeast)

**PATHOGENICITY:**   Causes protothecosis, which may be cutaneous, subcutaneous, or systemic. Infection may arise through traumatic implantation into subcutaneous tissue. The organism has also been isolated from clinical specimens in the absence of disease.

**RATE OF GROWTH:**   Rapid; mature in 3 days.

**COLONY MORPHOLOGY:**   Dull white to cream colored; yeastlike in consistency.

**MICROSCOPIC MORPHOLOGY:**   Sporangia of various sizes (6–26 µm in diameter) containing sporangiospores (endospores). Budding does not occur; no hyphae are produced. The cells of *P. wickerhamii* are somewhat smaller than those of *P. zopfii*. *P. stagnora* produces a capsule.
See Tables 4.1 (p. 64) and 4.4 (p. 79) for identification of yeastlike organisms.

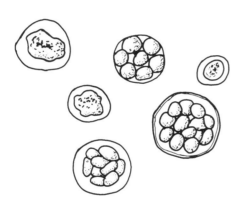
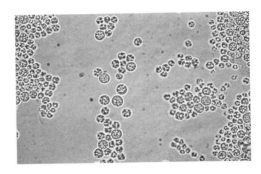

*For further information, see*
  *Kwon-Chung and Bennett, 1992, pp. 785–794*
  *McGinnis, 1980, p. 394*
  *Rippon, 1988, pp. 723–728*

# Blastoschizomyces capitatus (formerly Trichosporon capitatum)

**PATHOGENICITY:** Infrequent cause of invasive, systemic infection in immuno-compromised hosts, most commonly in neutropenic leukemia patients. Lesions have occurred in the lung, kidney, liver, spleen, brain, and other organs; it has also caused endocarditis. The organism is distributed in nature and may be found as normal flora of the skin, respiratory tract, and gastrointestinal tract.

**RATE OF GROWTH:** Rapid; mature in 5 days.

**COLONY MORPHOLOGY:** Yeastlike, smooth to wrinkled, radiating edges, developing short aerial hyphae with age; white to cream colored.

**MICROSCOPIC MORPHOLOGY:** On cornmeal-Tween 80 agar, round to oval budding yeastlike cells, hyphae and pseudohyphae, few arthroconidia in young colonies, and many annelloconidia are seen. Annellides form along the hyphae or at the ends of hyphal branches; annelloconidia are oblong and accumulate in clusters at the tips of the annellides. It is difficult to determine that the conidia are annelloconidia and not arthroconidia or blastoconidia; this accounts for its confusion with (and sometimes misidentification as) *Trichosporon beigelii* or *Candida krusei*. Careful attention to biochemical test results is required to differentiate these organisms. See Table 4.2 (p. 66) and Table 4.4 (p. 79).

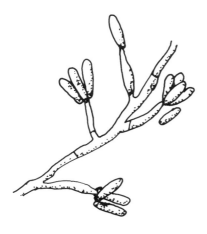
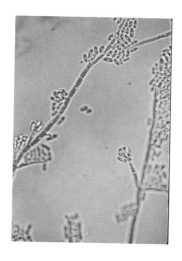

*For further information, see*
  *Kwon-Chung and Bennett, 1992, pp. 768–771*
  *Salkin et al., 1985a*
  *Polacheck et al., 1992*

## *Trichosporon* spp.

(This genus is currently undergoing taxonomic reevaluation; previously accepted nomenclature will be used in this guide until the issue is settled.)

**PATHOGENICITY:**   *Trichosporon beigelii* is increasingly involved in invasive localized and disseminated disease. Infection may be superficial, subcutaneous, or systemic. Immunocompromised patients with neutropenia are especially susceptible. *T. beigelii* classically causes white piedra, a superficial infection of the hair characterized by relatively soft, white nodules located along the shafts of hair. (Black piedra is caused by *Piedraia hortae*, p. 142.) White piedra usually involves the hairs of the beard and mustache, but may also infect the hairs on the scalp and pubic region. Several species of this genus, including *T. beigelii*, are also found as normal flora in the skin, nails, and mouth.

**RATE OF GROWTH:**   Rapid; mature in 5 days.

**COLONY MORPHOLOGY:**   Yeastlike; at first cream colored, moist, and soft, later it is finely wrinkled and more adherent to agar, the center becomes heaped, and the color darkens to become yellowish gray.

**MICROSCOPIC MORPHOLOGY:**   On cornmeal-Tween 80 agar at 25°C for 72 h, true hyphae and pseudohyphae with blastoconidia singly or in short chains are seen. Arthroconidia (2–4 × 3–9 µm) form on older cultures. The presence of blastoconidia along the hyphae differentiates *Trichosporon* from *Geotrichum* spp.

See Tables 4.1 (p. 64) and 4.4 (p. 79) for further differentiation of yeastlike organisms.

*Note*: Because of shared antigens, sera from patients with disseminated *T. beigelii* infection may give positive reactions with the cryptococcal latex test.

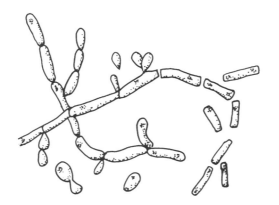 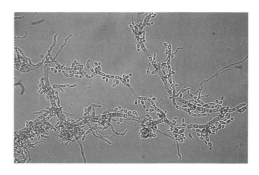

For further information, see
    Kwon-Chung and Bennett, 1992, pp. 183–190, 774–778
    Rippon, 1988, pp. 163–168, 611–615

**PATHOGENICITY:** Causes geotrichosis, which is a rare infection that is known to have produced lesions in the lungs, mouth, intestines, vagina, and skin. Fungemia and disseminated infection have also been reported. *Geotrichum* is found as normal flora in humans and seems to cause disease only in compromised hosts.

**RATE OF GROWTH:** Rapid; mature in 4 days.

**COLONY MORPHOLOGY:** At 25°C, young colonies are white, moist, yeastlike, and easily picked up. Submerged hyphae are later seen at the periphery, giving the appearance of ground glass. Some strains develop a short, white, cottony, aerial mycelium. Most strains do not grow at 37°C, but some may have a small amount of surface growth and extensive subsurface growth at this temperature.

**MICROSCOPIC MORPHOLOGY:** Coarse true hyphae (no pseudohyphae) that segment into rectangular arthroconidia which vary in length (4–10 μm) and in the roundness of their ends. Some may become quite round. The rectangular cells characteristically germinate from one corner. The absence of blastoconidia along the hyphae differentiates this organism from *Trichosporon* spp. (p. 88), and the consecutive formation of the arthroconidia serves to separate it from *Coccidioides immitis* (p. 186).

See Tables 4.1 (p. 64) and 4.4 (p. 79) for differentiation of yeastlike organisms.

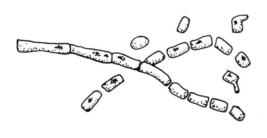 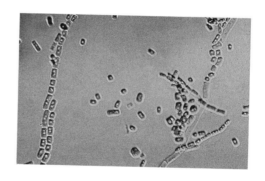

*For further information, see*
  *Kwon-Chung and Bennett, 1992, pp. 740–743*
  *McGinnis, 1980, pp. 221–225*
  *Rippon, 1988, pp. 714–718*

# ■ Thermally Dimorphic Fungi

# 5

The fungi included here are unique in that they grow as filamentous molds when cultured on routine mycology agar, such as Sabouraud dextrose agar, at 25–30°C and are yeastlike when cultured on brain heart infusion agar at 35–37°C. All of them are known to be pathogenic.

*Coccidioides immitis* (often placed with these organisms in other texts) does *NOT* produce yeastlike colonies or cells at 35–37°C on routine mycology agar; therefore, in this guide it is placed with the hyaline hyphomycetes (p. 186).

*Cokeromyces recurvatus* is thermally dimorphic, but because of its zygomycetous properties, it has been placed with that class (p. 115).

*For further information, see*
  *Murray et al., 1995, Manual of Clinical Microbiology, 6th ed., chapter 62*

**PATHOGENICITY:**   Causes sporotrichosis, a chronic infection that frequently begins as a lesion of the skin and subcutaneous tissue and then involves the lymphatic channels and lymph nodes draining the area. The disease may become systemic, disseminating most commonly to the skeletal system. Primary pulmonary sporotrichosis occurs with prevalence among chronic alcoholics.

**RATE OF GROWTH:**   Rapid; mature in 4 days.

**COLONY MORPHOLOGY:**   Thermally dimorphic. At 25–30°C the colonies are at first small and white with no cottony aerial hyphae. Later, colonies become moist, wrinkled, leathery, or velvety and often darken to brown or black. Some isolates are black from the beginning; stock cultures may remain nonpigmented.

At 35–37°C, colonies are cream or tan, smooth, and yeastlike. It is best to use brain heart infusion agar and transfer several generations to get a good yeast phase (p. 220).

**MICROSCOPIC MORPHOLOGY:**   At 25–30°C, hyphae are thin (1–2 μm in diameter), septate, and branching, with slender, tapering conidiophores rising at right angles. The apex of the conidiophore is often slightly swollen and bears many small pear-shaped or almost round conidia (2–3 × 3–6 μm) on delicate threadlike denticles, forming a "rosette"-like cluster in young cultures; conidia are later found singly along the conidiophores and hyphae.

At 35–37°C, round, oval, and fusiform budding cells of various sizes (1–3 × 3–10 μm), commonly called "cigar bodies," are seen.

The conversion of the mycelial form to the yeastlike form is essential for identification (see p. 220).

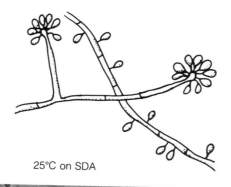

25°C on SDA

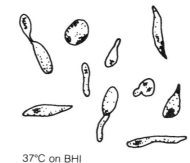

37°C on BHI

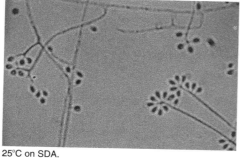

25°C on SDA.

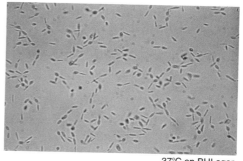

37°C on BHI agar.

*For further information, see*
*Evans and Richardson, 1989, pp. 134–137*
*Kwon-Chung and Bennett, 1992, pp. 707–729*
*McGinnis, 1980, pp. 278–279, 514–515*
*Rippon, 1988, pp. 325–352*
*Wentworth, 1988, pp. 99–106*

**PATHOGENICITY:** Causes histoplasmosis, which may be an acute, benign pulmonary disease or may be chronic or progressive and fatal. It may be localized or cause a disseminated infection, primarily of the reticuloendothelial system, and involve various tissues and organs of the body.

**RATE OF GROWTH:** Slow; mycelial forms usually mature within 15–20 days but may take up to 8 weeks. (The organism does not survive well in clinical specimens, so when histoplasmosis is suspected, the specimen must be processed immediately.)

**COLONY MORPHOLOGY:** Thermally dimorphic. At 25–30°C on Sabouraud dextrose agar (SDA), it is white to brown, or pinkish, with a fine, dense cottony texture. The reverse is white, sometimes yellow or orange tan. Brain heart infusion (BHI) agar may be the best growth medium, but characteristic morphology of the mold phase is seen on SDA.

At 35–37°C on BHI agar, moist, white, yeastlike colonies may eventually form, often requiring many generations. The yeast phase is inhibited by cycloheximide.

**MICROSCOPIC MORPHOLOGY:** At 25–30°C, in young cultures, septate hyphae are seen bearing round to pear-shaped, smooth or occasionally spiny microconidia (2–5 µm in diameter) on short branches or directly on the sides of the hyphae. At this early stage it can be confused with *Blastomyces* spp. (p. 96). After several weeks, large, thick-walled, round to pear-shaped tuberculate, knobby macroconidia (7–15 µm in diameter) are formed; these resemble the conidia of *Sepedonium* sp. (p. 205). Occasionally the walls of the macroconidia may be smooth.

At 35–37°C, small, round or oval budding cells (2–3 × 4–5 µm) and occasional abortive hyphae may be seen.

The conversion of the mycelial form to the yeast phase has been required in the past for morphologic identification (see p. 220) but is not always possible in vitro. A test for specific exoantigen or commercially available DNA probe analysis can more readily be used to confirm the identification.

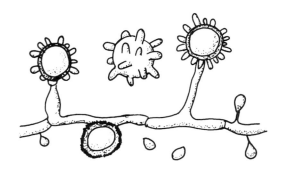

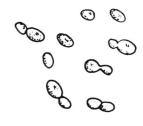

25°C on SDA

37°C on BHI

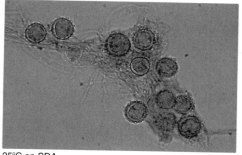

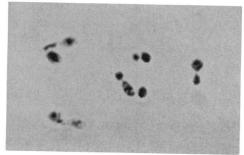

25°C on SDA.

37°C on BHI agar.

For further information, see
  Evans and Richardson, 1989, pp. 144–148
  Kwon-Chung and Bennett, 1992, pp. 464–513
  McGinnis, 1980, pp. 229–231, 500–504
  Rippon, 1988, pp. 381–423
  Wentworth, 1988, pp. 206–215

**PATHOGENICITY:** Causes blastomycosis, which is a chronic infection characterized by suppurative and granulomatous lesions in any part of the body; it most commonly begins in the lungs and is disseminated to the skin and bones.

**RATE OF GROWTH:** Slow; mycelial forms mature within 14 days. Some strains are slower; cultures should be held for 8 weeks if blastomycosis is suspected. (Organism does not survive well in specimens and must therefore be cultured immediately.)

**COLONY MORPHOLOGY:** Thermally dimorphic. At 25–30°C on Sabouraud dextrose agar (SDA), it is at first yeastlike, then prickly, and finally very cottony with a white aerial mycelium; it turns tan or brown with age. Reverse is tan.

At 35–37°C, it is cream to tan in color, heaped or wrinkled, and waxy in appearance; it is best seen on brain heart infusion (BHI) agar. Yeast phase is inhibited by cycloheximide.

**MICROSCOPIC MORPHOLOGY:** At 25–30°C on SDA, it forms septate hyphae bearing round or pear-shaped conidia (2–10 μm in diameter) attached to conidiophores of various lengths or directly on the hyphae. May resemble *Scedosporium apiospermum* (p. 132) or *Chrysosporium* spp. (p. 203). Older cultures have thick-walled chlamydoconidia.

At 35–37°C on BHI agar, yeastlike cells (8–15 μm in diameter), budding on a broad base (4–5 μm wide), thick walled, and appearing double contoured, are seen.

Conversion from the mold to yeast phase is essential for identification (see p. 220). Testing with a nucleic acid probe or for exoantigen may also be used for confirmation of identification.

25°C on SDA

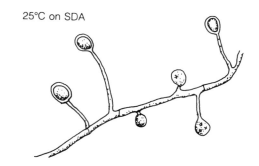

37°C on BHI

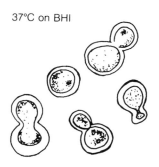

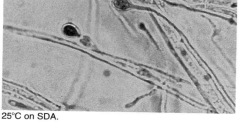

25°C on SDA.

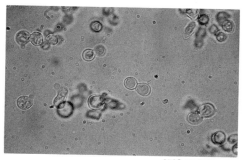

37°C on BHI agar.

For further information, see
Evans and Richardson, 1989, pp. 141–144
Kwon-Chung and Bennett, 1992, pp. 248–279
McGinnis, 1980, pp. 187–192, 477–480
Rippon, 1988, pp. 474–505
Wentworth, 1988, pp. 183–196

**PATHOGENICITY:** Causes paracoccidioidomycosis (South American blastomycosis), a chronic granulomatous disease characteristically beginning in the lungs and spreading to the mucous membranes of the nose, mouth, and occasionally the gastrointestinal tract. Dissemination to skin, lymph nodes, and other internal organs is common.

**RATE OF GROWTH:** Very slow; mycelial forms mature within 21 days.

**COLONY MORPHOLOGY:** Thermally dimorphic. At 25–30°C on Sabouraud dextrose agar (SDA), colony is white, heaped, compact, usually folded, and almost glabrous or with a short nap of white aerial mycelium that often turns brown with age.

At 35–37°C on brain heart infusion (BHI) agar, colony is heaped, cream to tan, moist, and soft, becoming waxy and yeastlike.

**MICROSCOPIC MORPHOLOGY:** At 25–30°C on SDA, usually only septate, branched hyphae with some intercalary and terminal chlamydospores are formed; a few microconidia are sometimes observed along the hyphae.

At 35–37°C on BHI agar, large, round, fairly thick-walled cells (5–50 μm) with single and multiple buddings (1–10 μm) are seen. The buds are attached to the mother cell by narrow connections and may almost completely surround the cell, giving the characteristic ship's wheel appearance. Care must be taken not to confuse single-budding cells with *Blastomyces dermatitidis*.

Conversion of the mold form to the yeast phase is essential for identification (see p. 220).

## *Paracoccidioides brasiliensis* (continued)

25°C on SDA

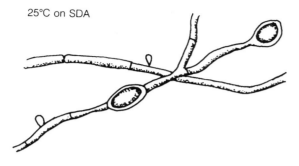

37°C on BHI

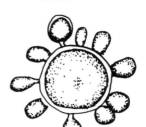

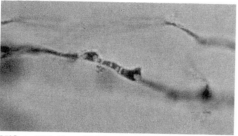

25°C on PDA. From Walsh et al., Manual of Clinical Microbiology, 6th ed.

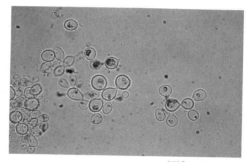

37°C on BHI agar.

*For further information, see*
*Evans and Richardson, 1989, pp. 151–153*
*Kwon-Chung and Bennett, 1992, pp. 594–619*
*McGinnis, 1980, pp. 248–251, 509–510*
*Rippon, 1988, pp. 506–531*
*Wentworth, 1988, pp. 215–219*

**PATHOGENICITY:** Causes deep-seated infection that can be focal or disseminated in both immunocompromised and apparently immunocompetent individuals who have traveled or lived in areas of Southeast Asia in which *P. marneffei* is endemic. Infections are being seen with increasing frequency in AIDS patients who have been in that area. The organism has been isolated from blood, bone marrow, skin, lung, mucosa, lymph nodes, urine, stool, cerebrospinal fluid, and various internal organs.

**RATE OF GROWTH:** Rapid; mature within 3 days at 25–30°C. Yeast form develops more slowly at 35–37°C. Sabouraud dextrose agar (SDA) supports growth at 25–37°C and demonstrates thermal dimorphism. Cycloheximide inhibits growth.

**COLONY MORPHOLOGY:** Thermally dimorphic. At 25–30°C on SDA, colony is flat, powdery to velvety, and tan, later becoming reddish yellow with a yellow or white edge; sometimes it is bluish gray-green in the center. A deep reddish soluble pigment diffuses into the medium after 3–7 days (other species of *Penicillium* may also produce a red pigment). Reverse is brownish red.

At 35–37°C on SDA, inhibitory mold agar (IMA), or brain heart infusion (BHI) agar, colony is soft, white to tan, dry, and yeastlike. Conversion from mycelial to yeast form may take up to 14 days; it is most rapidly accomplished (in approximately 4 days) by culturing in BHI broth on a shaker; the next best method is on 5% sheep blood agar.

**MICROSCOPIC MORPHOLOGY:** At 25–30°C, structures typical of the genus *Penicillium* (p. 193) develop, i.e., smooth conidiophores with terminal verticils of 4 to 5 metulae, each metula bearing 4 to 6 phialides. Conidia are smooth or slightly rough and oval (3–4 × 6–7 µm) and form chains; short, narrow extensions connect the conidia.

At 35–37°C, round or oval yeastlike cells (3–8 µm in length) are seen; central cross wall forms, as the cells multiply by fission rather than by budding.

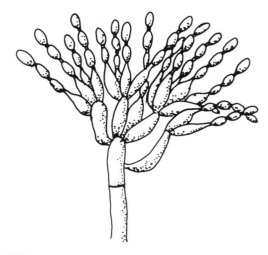

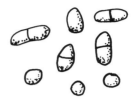

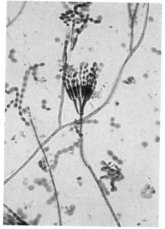

25°C on SDA. Courtesy of William Merz.

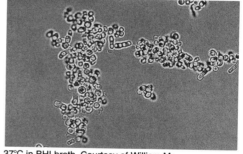

37°C in BHI broth. Courtesy of William Merz.

*For further information, see*
    *Hilmarsdottir et al., 1993*
    *Kwon-Chung and Bennett, 1992, pp. 755–758*
    *McGinnis, 1994*

# Thermally Monomorphic Molds

6

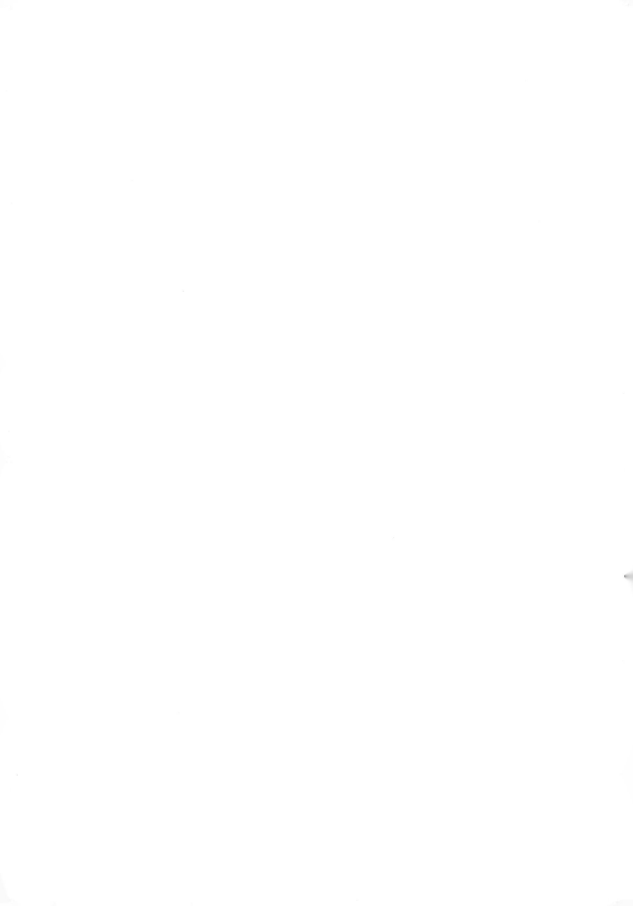

# ▉ Zygomycetes

Zygomycetes are a class of fungi that have broad hyphae (6–15 μm wide) and are almost nonseptate. Septa are most often seen on sporangiophores just below the sporangia and elsewhere in older cultures. Asexual reproduction occurs in a sac-like structure called a sporangium, in which the internal contents are cleaved into spores.

Most zygomycetes that are encountered in the clinical laboratory belong to the order Mucorales. These are easily recognized by their grayish, very fluffy colonies that rapidly fill the tube or petri plate in a cotton candy-like fashion. The differentiation of the various genera is based on:

1. The presence and location (or absence) of rhizoids (root-like structures along the vegetative hyphae);
2. The branching or unbranched nature of the sporangiophores (the stalks bearing the sac-like sporangia);
3. The shape of the columella (the small dome-like area at the apex of the sporangiophore);
4. The appearance of an apophysis (a broadening near the apex of the sporangiophore, just below the columella);
5. The size and shape of the sporangium (sac-like structure in which the spores are formed).

See labelled diagram, p. 111.

A few genera (*Apophysomyces* and *Saksenaea*) require special media (p. 220) to enhance sporulation.

Some of the Zygomycetes in the order Mucorales can cause severe disease (zygomycosis), predominantly in patients who are predisposed by diabetes, leukopenia, immunosuppression, AIDS, severe burns, intravenous drug abuse, malnutrition, etc. Infections have been reported from a wide range of anatomic sites but are most commonly rhinocerebral, pulmonary, cutaneous, and disseminated. The organisms are known for their disastrous ability to invade and block blood vessels.

The other order of Zygomycetes, the Entomophthorales, are less commonly encountered. Their colonies are flat and buff to grayish brown with a waxy texture, and they develop short aerial hyphae and darken with age. They have broad hyphae and unique microscopic structures. Two genera of Entomorphthorales (*Basidiobolus* and *Conidiobolus*) cause tropical subcutaneous mycoses and are discussed in the latter portion of this section.

*For further information, see*
  *Murray et al., 1995, Manual of Clinical Microbiology, 6th ed., chapter 65*

**PATHOGENICITY:** Occasionally the etiologic agent of zygomycosis (for description of disease see p. 106). This fungus is also known as a common contaminant.

**RATE OF GROWTH:** Rapid; mature within 4 days. Growth is inhibited by cycloheximide. Most species do not grow well at 37°C.

**COLONY MORPHOLOGY:** Quickly covers agar surface with fluff resembling cotton candy; white, later turns gray. Reverse is white.

**MICROSCOPIC MORPHOLOGY:** Hyphae are wide (6–15 μm) and practically non-septate. Sporangiophores are long and often branched and bear terminal round, spore-filled sporangia (50–300 μm in diameter). The sporangial wall dissolves, scattering the round or slightly oblong spores (4–8 μm in diameter), revealing the columella and sometimes leaving a collarette at the base of the sporangium. No rhizoids are formed.

See Table 6.1 (p. 109) for differentiation of similar organisms in the class Zygomycetes.

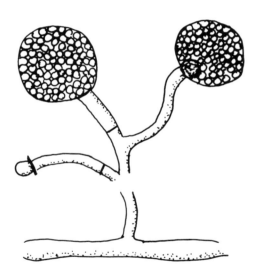
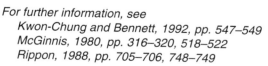
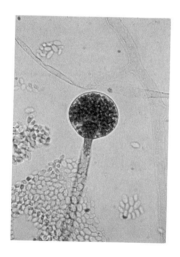

*For further information, see*
  *Kwon-Chung and Bennett, 1992, pp. 547–549*
  *McGinnis, 1980, pp. 316–320, 518–522*
  *Rippon, 1988, pp. 705–706, 748–749*

**PATHOGENICITY:**  Some species have been found to be etiologic agents of zygomycosis (see p. 106 for description of disease). They are also known as common contaminants.

**RATE OF GROWTH:**  Rapid; mature within 4 days. The pathogenic species grow well at 37°C. Growth is inhibited by cycloheximide.

**COLONY MORPHOLOGY:**  Quickly covers agar surface with dense growth that is cotton candy-like; colonies are at first white and then gray or yellowish brown. Reverse is white.

**MICROSCOPIC MORPHOLOGY:**  Broad hyphae (6–15 μm in diameter) have no, or very few, septa. Numerous stolons run among the mycelia, connecting groups of long sporangiophores that usually are unbranched. At the point where the stolons and sporangiophores meet, root-like hyphae (rhizoids) are produced. The sporangiophores are long (up to 4 mm) and terminate with a dark, round sporangium (40–350 μm in diameter) containing a columella and many oval, colorless or brown spores (4–11 μm). No collarette remains when the sporangial wall dissolves. This genus is differentiated from *Mucor* spp. (p. 107) by the presence of stolons, rhizoids, and usually unbranched sporangiophores. It is differentiated from *Absidia* spp. (p. 111) by the location of the rhizoids in relation to the sporangiophores and by the shape and size of the sporangia.

See Table 6.1 (p. 109) and Table 6.2 (p. 109) for identification of genus and species.

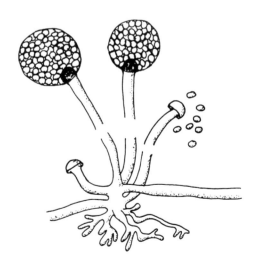

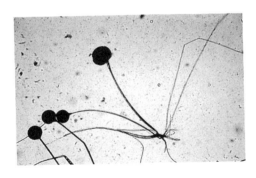

*For further information, see*
  *Evans and Richardson, 1989, pp. 154, 156*
  *Kwon-Chung and Bennett, 1992, pp. 541–545*
  *McGinnis, 1980, pp. 323–325, 518–522*
  *Rippon, 1988, pp. 702–705, 748–750*

**TABLE 6.1** Differential characteristics of similar organisms in the class *Zygomycetes*[a]

| Genus | Rhizoids | Sporangiophores | Apophysis | Columellae | Sporangia | Maximum growth temp (°C) |
|---|---|---|---|---|---|---|
| *Rhizopus* | Present | Single or in tufts; usually unbranched; mostly brown | Mostly inconspicuous | Almost round or slightly elongated | Round | ~45 |
| *Rhizomucor* | Present | Branched; dark brown | Absent (or very tiny) | Almost round | Round | ~54 |
| *Mucor* | Absent | Branched or unbranched, mostly hyaline | Absent | Various shapes | Round | <37 |
| *Absidia* | Present, but often indistinct | Finely branched; almost hyaline | Conspicuous, conical | Semicircle, may have projection at top | Pyriform (pear shaped) | ~45 |
| *Apophysomyces* | Present | Generally single and unbranched; grayish brown | Conspicuous, bell shaped | Semicircle, may be elongated | Pyriform | ≥42 |

[a] Adapted from Scholer et al. (1983), with additions.

**TABLE 6.2** Differential characteristics of the clinically encountered *Rhizopus* spp.[a]

| Organism | Pathogenic | Maximum growth temp (°C) | Rhizoid length (µm) | Sporangiophore length (µm) | Sporangium diameter (µm) | Columellae | Sporangiospores |
|---|---|---|---|---|---|---|---|
| *R. oryzae* (arrhizus) (most common agent of zygomycosis) | + | 40–46 | 150–300 | 500–3,500 | 50–250 | Almost round | Variable size, average length 6–8 µm; striated; elongate to lemon shaped |
| *R. microsporus* var. *rhizopodiformis* | + | 50–52 | 100–120 | 200–1,000 | 40–130 | Slightly elongated; distinct apophysis | Equal in size, average length 4–6 µm; smooth to slightly striated; almost round to slightly elongated |
| *R. stolonifer* | 0 | 30–32 | 300–350 | 1,500–4,000 | 150–350 | Almost round | Variable in size, average length, 9–11 µm; very striated; elongate to polyhedric |

[a] Abbreviations: +, positive; 0, negative.

**PATHOGENICITY:** An etiologic agent of zygomycosis (for description of disease, see p. 106). Incidence in the clinical laboratory is uncertain, as isolates in the past have probably been misidentified.

**RATE OF GROWTH:** Rapid; mature within 4 days. Members of the genus are thermophilic; maximum growth temperature is 54–58°C. Growth is inhibited by cycloheximide.

**COLONY MORPHOLOGY:** Very fluffy growth with texture of cotton candy; gray, becoming dark brown with age. Reverse is white.

**MICROSCOPIC MORPHOLOGY:** Appears to be intermediate between *Rhizopus* (p. 108) and *Mucor* (p. 107) spp. Sporangia are round and are usually 60–100 μm in diameter. A few primitive, short, irregularly branched rhizoids are formed, differentiating the organism from *Mucor* spp. It differs from *Rhizopus* spp. by having branched sporangiophores and by the location of the rhizoids (at points on the stolon between the sporangiophores).

See Table 6.1 (p. 109) for differentiation of similar organisms in the class Zygomycetes.

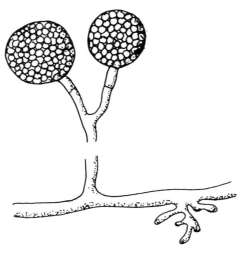
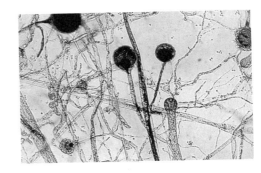

*For further information, see*
*Evans and Richardson, 1989, pp. 154–157*
*Kwon-Chung and Bennett, 1992, pp. 546, 549*
*McGinnis, 1980, pp. 321–322, 518–522*
*Rippon, 1988, p. 706*

**PATHOGENICITY:** An infrequent etiologic agent of zygomycosis (for description of disease, see p. 106). The organism is ubiquitous and may therefore be a contaminant in cultures.

**RATE OF GROWTH:** Rapid; mature within 4 days. Growth is inhibited by cycloheximide.

**COLONY MORPHOLOGY:** Coarse wooly gray surface; rapidly covers agar slant with fluff resembling gray cotton candy. Reverse is white.

**MICROSCOPIC MORPHOLOGY:** Hyphae are wide (6–15 µm in diameter) and nonseptate (or almost so). It is similar in structure to *Rhizopus* spp. (p. 108) except that the sporangiophores of *Absidia* arise at points on the stolon that are between the rhizoids and not opposite them. Also, the sporangiophores (up to 450 µm long) are branched and widen, forming a conical apophysis just below the columella. The columella is typically shaped like a semicircle with a small projection on top. The sporangia are relatively small (20–120 µm in diameter) and slightly pear shaped instead of spherical. When the sporangial wall dissolves, a short collarette often remains where the wall met the sporangiophore. The sporangiospores are round to oval (3–4.5 µm).

*Note:* The rhizoids may be difficult to find and are best observed by using a dissecting microscope to examine colonies on an agar surface.

See Table 6.1 (p. 109) for differentiation of similar organisms in the class Zygomycetes.

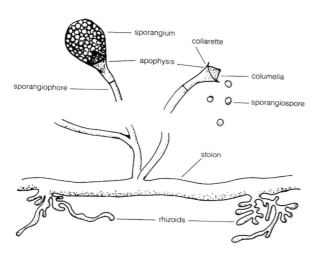
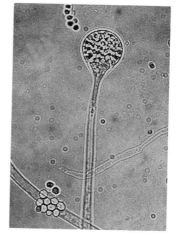

*For further information, see*
  *Kwon-Chung and Bennett, 1992, pp. 544–548*
  *McGinnis, 1980, pp. 304–306, 518–522*
  *Rippon, 1988, pp. 706–707, 751–752*

**PATHOGENICITY:**   Occasional agent of zygomycosis. Infection is acquired by traumatic implantation such as accidental injuries, surgery, insect bites, and contamination of burns. Most infected patients appear to be otherwise immunocompetent. The organism is found in soil.

**RATE OF GROWTH:**   Rapid; growth fills plate/tube within 4 days; grows at temperatures up to 42°C. It grows on media containing cycloheximide (in contrast to other zygomycetes).

**COLONY MORPHOLOGY:**   Fluffy cottony growth that fills tube or plate; surface is white when young, becoming cream to yellow or brownish gray with age. Reverse is white to pale yellow.

**MICROSCOPIC MORPHOLOGY:**   Sporulation does not occur on routine media; only broad, almost nonseptate hyphae form. A special culture method (p. 220) is required to induce sporulation. Hyphae are generally nonseptate and branched (4–8 μm in diameter). Sporangiophores are long (up to 530 μm) and unbranched and arise singly from a hyphal segment that resembles the foot cells seen in *Aspergillus* spp. (p. 192); the apex of the sporangiophore widens to form a funnel-shaped or bell-shaped apophysis (11–40 μm in diameter at the widest part). The columella is a half circle. Sporangia are pear shaped/pyriform (20–58 μm in diameter) and upon dissolution may leave a small collar at the base of the columella. The sporangiospores are smooth and mostly oblong (5–8 μm in length) and may appear pale brown in mass. Rhizoids may be between the points of origin of the sporangiophores or opposite the sporangiophore, depending on the media.
　　*Apophysomyces* is similar to *Absidia* but differs by having:

A more pronounced apophysis which is bell shaped rather than conical;
A "foot cell" at the base of the sporangiophore;
Sporangiophores developing opposite rhizoids on plain agar;
Darkening and thickening of the sporangiophore wall below the apophysis;
Failure to sporulate readily with routine culture methods.

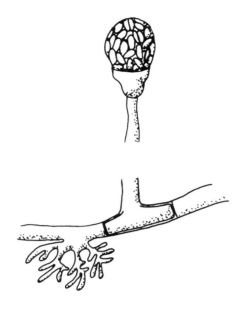

Courtesy of Ira Salkin.

*For further information, see*
  *Kwon-Chung and Bennett, 1992, p. 550*
  *Misra et al., 1979*

**PATHOGENICITY:** Occasionally an agent of zygomycosis. Cases are usually preceded by traumatic implantation. Infections have included rhinocerebral, cranial, osteomyelitic, cutaneous, and subcutaneous lesions. Many of the patients appear to be otherwise immunocompetent.

**RATE OF GROWTH:** Rapid; growth fills plate/tube within 4 days. Maximum growth temperature is 44°C.

**COLONY MORPHOLOGY:** Very cottony, fluffy white surface. Reverse is white.

**MICROSCOPIC MORPHOLOGY:** On routine media the organism does not sporulate; only broad, mostly nonseptate, branched, hyaline hyphae form. A special procedure (p. 220) is required for stimulation of sporulation. Sporangiophores (24–64 µm long) bear sporangia that are flask shaped (50–150 µm long), having a swollen portion near the base and a long neck that broadens at the apex. Sporangiospores are elongate (3–4 µm long) and smooth. Rhizoids form near the base of the sporangiophore, are dichotomously branched, and darken with age.

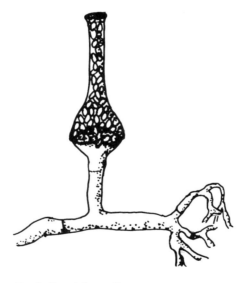
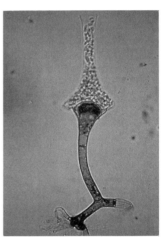

Courtesy of Ira Salkin.

*For further information, see*
   *Kwon-Chung and Bennett, 1992, pp. 528, 534–535, 551*

**PATHOGENICITY:** The organism has been recovered several times from genito-urinary sites (cervix, vagina, bladder), but there was no tissue invasion demonstrated. It appears to have a predilection for colonization of those sites; its possible role as an etiologic agent of mycotic disease is uncertain.

**RATE OF GROWTH:** Moderate; mature in 5 to 10 days.

**COLONY MORPHOLOGY:** At 25–30°C on Sabouraud dextrose agar, thermally dimorphic colonies are tan, thin, and radially wrinkled, with central areas becoming gray; entire colony becomes brown with age. Reverse is tan to brown.

At 35–37°C on enriched medium such as brain heart infusion agar, preferably in 5–7% $CO_2$, tan to gray slightly wrinkled yeastlike colonies develop in 2 days.

**MICROSCOPIC MORPHOLOGY:** At 25–30°C, broad, sparsely septate hyphae are seen. Sporangiophores (100–500 μm long) terminate in a round vesicle that produces recurving stalks, each bearing a round sporangiole (9–13 μm in diameter). The sporangiole contains 12–20 sporangiospores that are smooth walled and of variable size and shape, mostly oval (average, 2.5 × 4.5 μm). Zygospores are abundantly produced between pairs of hyphal segments, sporangiophores, or suspensors of mature zygospores. Mature zygospores are round (35–55 μm in diameter), brown, rough walled; the organism is homothallic, i.e., it requires only one thallus for production of sexual spores. No rhizoids are formed.

At 35–37°C in 5–7% $CO_2$, thin-walled, round yeast cells (15–90 μm in diameter) develop, with single or multiple budding that may resemble the "ship's wheel" appearance of *Paracoccidioides brasiliensis* (p. 98).

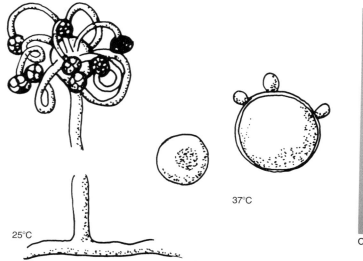

25°C

37°C

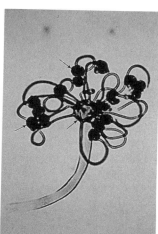

Courtesy of Ira Salkin.

*For further information, see*
*Kemna et al., 1994*
*McGough et al., 1990*

**PATHOGENICITY:**  Commonly considered a contaminant, but has been involved in a few disseminated and pulmonary infections in compromised hosts.

**RATE OF GROWTH:**  Rapid; mature within 4 days. Growth is inhibited by cycloheximide.

**COLONY MORPHOLOGY:**  Very fluffy, like cotton candy; white, then gray. Reverse is white.

**MICROSCOPIC MORPHOLOGY:**  Broad hyphae, almost nonseptate. Sporangiophores are long, branched, ending in swollen vesicles (30–65 μm in diameter). The vesicles are covered with spine-like denticles, each supporting a round to oval sporangiolum (5–8 × 6–14 μm). The walls of the sporangiola are often encrusted with needle-like crystals.

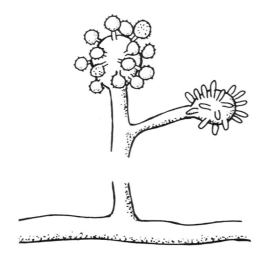 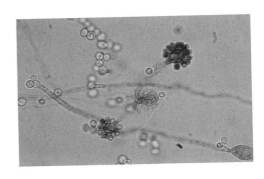

For further information, see
   Kwon-Chung and Bennett, 1992, pp. 550–551, 802
   McGinnis, 1980, pp. 313, 315, 318
   Rippon, 1988, pp. 684, 752, 754

**PATHOGENICITY:** Considered a contaminant; very rarely involved in infection.

**RATE OF GROWTH:** Rapid; mature within 3 days.

**COLONY MORPHOLOGY:** Quickly fills petri plate with white cotton candy-like fluff, then turns dark gray to almost black. Reverse is white.

**MICROSCOPIC MORPHOLOGY:** Hyphae are broad (4–8 μm in diameter) and almost nonseptate (irregular septa may form with age). Has sporangiophores that are rather short and branched and have very swollen tips. On the enlarged round tip of the sporangiophore are chains of round spores enclosed in finger-like tubular sporangia (4–6 × 9–60 μm). Rhizoids are usually formed. This organism may at first resemble *Aspergillus niger* (p. 190), but careful examination reveals the tubular sporangia and the absence of phialides.

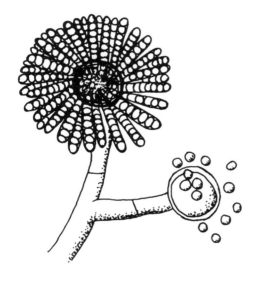
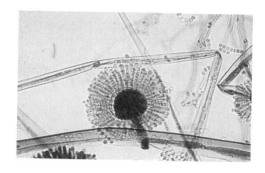

*For further information, see*
  *Kwon-Chung and Bennett, 1992, pp. 551–552, 807*
  *McGinnis, 1980, pp. 324–326*
  *Rippon, 1988, p. 751*

**PATHOGENICITY:** Etiologic agent of entomophthoromycosis basidiobolae (subcutaneous zygomycosis), which is a chronic inflammatory or granulomatous disease generally restricted to the limbs, chest, back, or buttocks. The lesions are characteristically huge, palpable, hard, nonulcerating subcutaneous masses. On rare occasions systemic infections have occurred.

**RATE OF GROWTH:** Rapid; mature within 5 days.

**COLONY MORPHOLOGY:** Thin, flat, waxy; buff to gray. Becomes heaped up or radially folded, grayish brown, and covered with white aerial hyphae. Reverse is white. Some strains have an earthy odor similar to that of *Streptomyces* spp.

**MICROSCOPIC MORPHOLOGY:** Wide (8–20 μm) hyphae having occasional septa that become numerous with the production of spores. Short sporophores enlarge apically to form a swollen area from which a single-celled spore and a fragment of the sporophore are forcibly discharged. Other sporophores (not swollen) passively release club-shaped spores having a knob-like tip and can function as sporangia. The organism also produces many round intercalary zygospores (20–50 μm in diameter) with smooth (occasionally rough), thick walls and a prominent beak-like appendage (remnant of a copulatory tube) on one side.

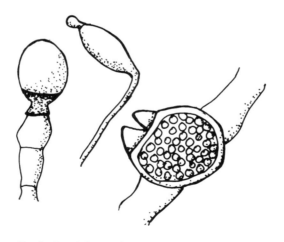 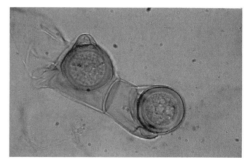

*For further information, see*
  *Kwon-Chung and Bennett, 1992, pp. 447–463*
  *McGinnis, 1980, pp. 306–309, 517*
  *Rippon, 1988, pp. 692–693, 708–709*
  *Wentworth, 1988, pp. 151–157, 225–227*

**PATHOGENICITY:** Etiologic agent of entomophthoromycosis conidiobolae, which is a chronic inflammatory or granulomatous disease usually restricted to the nasal mucosa; it can spread to adjacent subcutaneous tissue and cause disfigurement of the face. The disease is characterized by polyps or palpable subcutaneous masses. On rare occasion, this and other species of the genus have caused deeply invasive, life-threatening infections.

**RATE OF GROWTH:** Rapid; mature within 5 days.

**COLONY MORPHOLOGY:** Flat, waxy; buff or gray, becoming sparsely covered with short white aerial hyphae. With age, colony becomes tan to brown. Reverse is white. Sides of culture tube or plate become covered with spores forcibly discharged by the sporophores.

**MICROSCOPIC MORPHOLOGY:** Hyphae have few septa; unbranched sporophores bear single-celled round spores (10–30 μm in diameter). At maturity, the spores are forcibly ejected and bear a broad, tapering projection at the site of former attachment. The spores may germinate and produce long hyphal tubes that become sporophores, each bearing another spore. A spore may also develop a number of short extensions that give rise to a corona of secondary spores. Spores may produce short, hair-like appendages.

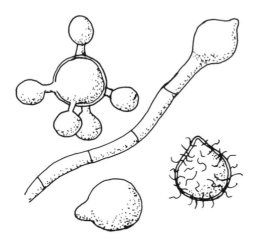

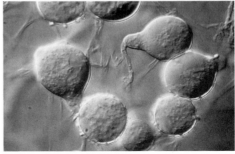

Courtesy of Michael McGinnis.

*For further information, see*
  *Kwon-Chung and Bennett, 1992, pp. 447–463*
  *McGinnis, 1980, pp. 310–313, 516–517*
  *Rippon, 1988, pp. 690–692, 709–710*
  *Walsh et al., 1994*
  *Wentworth, 1988, pp. 151–159, 225–226*

# ◾ Dematiaceous Fungi

Dematiaceous fungi include a large group of organisms that produce dark (olive, brown, gray, or black) colonies because of a melanin pigment in their cell walls.

The diseases produced by some of the dematiaceous fungi are classified according to the clinical presentation and the appearance of the organism in tissue:

1. Chromoblastomycosis: The fungi are seen in tissue as sclerotic bodies. These structures are round (5 to 12 μm in diameter), brownish, usually with a single septum or two intersecting septa. The infection is chronic and causes the development of warty nodules, tumor-like masses, or raised, rough, cauliflower-like lesions containing the sclerotic bodies. The lesions usually develop in the subcutaneous tissue of the lower extremities but are sometimes on other exposed areas such as the hands, head region, or trunk. On rare occasions, the etiologic agents have been known to spread to the central nervous system, lungs, or muscular tissues.

2. Phaeohyphomycosis: The etiologic agents occur in tissue as dark yeastlike cells, pseudohypha-like elements, variously shaped hyphae, or any combination of these forms. The infection may be cutaneous, subcutaneous, or systemic.

3. Mycetoma: The infection is chronic and characterized by swollen tumor-like lesions that yield granular pus through draining sinuses. The granules of eumycotic mycetoma contain variously shaped fungal elements (many of the etiologic agents are not de-

matiaceous). The infection occurs most often in the feet or hands but may occur on any exposed parts of the body.

Tinea nigra and black piedra are also caused by dematiaceous fungi.

Many of the infections caused by the dematiaceous fungi are due to traumatic implantation of the organism from the environment into cutaneous or subcutaneous tissue, but pulmonary or disseminated infections have been initiated by inhalation of conidia.

Although the dematiaceous fungi are not highly virulent, some are regularly seen as etiologic agents of disease while others usually are encountered as saprophytes or contaminants and only occasionally act as opportunistic pathogens.

*Sporothrix schenckii* grows as a dematiaceous fungus when incubated at 25–30°C, but it is yeastlike and nonpigmented at 35–37°C and therefore placed with the thermally dimorphic fungi (p. 92).

*For further information, see*
  *Murray et al., 1995, Manual of Clinical Microbiology, 6th ed., chapters 66 and 67*

**PATHOGENICITY:**  The most common worldwide cause of chromoblastomycosis (for description of disease, see p. 121). The lesions usually develop in the subcutaneous tissue on the lower extremities, but sometimes are on other exposed areas. On very rare occasion the organism has been known to cause internal infections.

**RATE OF GROWTH:**  Slow; mature in 14 days.

**COLONY MORPHOLOGY:**  Surface is dark green, gray, or black, covered with silvery, velvety mycelium; colonies are usually flat and then develop a convex cone-shaped protrusion in the center. Colony becomes slightly imbedded in the medium. Reverse is black.

**MICROSCOPIC MORPHOLOGY:**  Hyphae are septate, branched, and brown; conidia are dark, 1.5–3.0 × 2.5–6.0 µm. Conidiation is enhanced on cornmeal agar or potato dextrose agar. Four types of conidial formation may be seen:

1. *Fonsecaea* type: Conidiophores are septate, erect, and compactly sympodial. The distal end of the conidiophore develops swollen denticles that bear primary single-celled ovoid conidia. Denticles on the primary conidia support secondary single-celled conidia that may produce tertiary conidia, but long chains are not formed. Elongate conidia often form in verticils at fertile sites along the conidiophore forming an asterisk-like appearance.
2. *Rhinocladiella* type: Conidiophores are septate, erect, and sympodial; swollen denticles bear ovoid conidia at the tip and along the side of the conidiophore. Usually only primary conidia develop; secondary conidia are rare.
3. *Cladosporium* type: Conidiophores are erect and give rise to large primary shield-shaped conidia that in turn produce short, branching chains of oval conidia having small dark hila (scars of attachment).
4. *Phialophora* type: Phialides are vase shaped with terminal cuplike collarettes. Round to oval conidia accumulate at the apex of the phialide. This type of conidiation is often scant or lacking.

*Note*: In tissues, this organism, as well as the other etiologic agents of chromoblastomycosis, appears as large (5–12 µm in diameter), round, brownish, thick-walled cells with horizontal and vertical septa. When cultured at 25, 30, or 37°C, the organisms are filamentous.

*(continued on following page)*

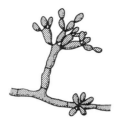
Fonsecaea-type
conidiation

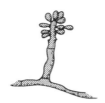
Rhinocladiella-type
conidiation

Phialophora-type
conidiation

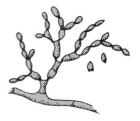
Cladosporium-type
conidiation

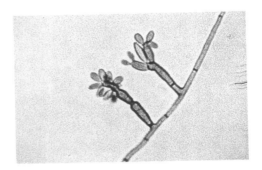

For further information, see
Kwon-Chung and Bennett, 1992, pp. 337–349
McGinnis, 1980, pp. 213–219, 482–484
Rippon, 1988, pp. 276, 287–293
Wentworth, 1988, pp. 117–128

**PATHOGENICITY:** Causes chromoblastomycosis. For description of disease, see p. 121. This organism is rarely encountered.

**RATE OF GROWTH:** Very slow; mature in 28 days.

**COLONY MORPHOLOGY:** Surface is dark green to black, heaped, and brittle, with irregular indented border. After 3 or 4 weeks, brownish hyphae appear on the surface with typical conidiophores and conidial formations. Reverse is black.

**MICROSCOPIC MORPHOLOGY:** On Sabouraud dextrose agar, hyphae are septate, brown, and branched and bear predominantly *Fonsecaea*-type conidiophores that produce short chains and masses of almost round conidia (1.5–3 μm in diameter). The outstanding characteristics of this species are (i) the cask-like shape of the conidia with the wide diameter of the septa between conidia, and (ii) the compact arrangement of the conidial chains that are not easily dissociated. *Rhinocladiella*-, *Cladosporium*-, and *Phialophora*-type conidiation (p. 123) may also be seen.

In tissue, the organisms appear as dark, round, septate cells (5–12 μm in diameter).

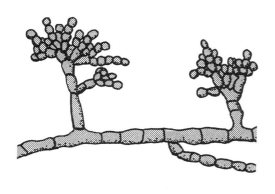

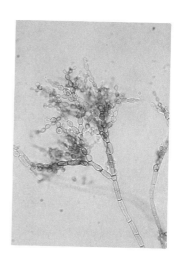

For further information, see
   Kwon-Chung and Bennett, 1992, pp. 349–350
   McGinnis, 1980, pp. 213–218, 221–222, 482–484
   Rippon, 1988, p. 293

**PATHOGENICITY:**   Causes chromoblastomycosis, of which it is the second most common etiologic agent worldwide (the most common in North America). It is also an etiologic agent of phaeohyphomycosis and, on rare occasion, mycetoma. For description of diseases, see p. 121.

**RATE OF GROWTH:**   Slow; mature in 14 days.

**COLONY MORPHOLOGY:**   Surface is dark greenish brown to black with a close matlike olive to gray mycelium. Some strains are heaped and granular; others are flat. Colonies become imbedded in the medium. Reverse is black.

**MICROSCOPIC MORPHOLOGY:**   Hyphae are brown, branched, and septate. Phialides are vase shaped with a flared cuplike collarette. Round to oval conidia (1–3 × 2–4 μm) accumulate at the apex of the phialide giving the appearance of a vase of flowers.

In tissue, the organism appears as dark, round, septate cells (5–12 μm in diameter).

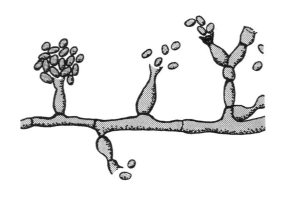 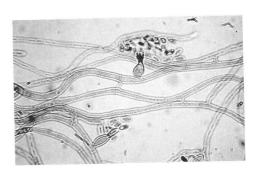

For further information, see
    Kwon-Chung and Bennett, 1992, pp. 346–347
    McGinnis, 1980, pp. 261–265, 482–484
    Rippon, 1988, pp. 293–294
For information on other species of Phialophora, see
    Dixon and Polak-Wyss, 1991

**PATHOGENICITY:** An etiologic agent of phaeohyphomycosis* (see p. 121 for description of disease).

**RATE OF GROWTH:** Moderate; mature in 5–7 days.

**COLONY MORPHOLOGY:** Surface is olive brown to brownish gray, wooly to velvety; brown diffusing pigment may develop with age. Reverse is dark.

**MICROSCOPIC MORPHOLOGY:** Septate hyphae are at first colorless and become brown. Phialides are slightly flask shaped with a characteristic flared, saucer-shaped collarette; simple, unflared phialides also form. Conidia are pale and oval or brown and round (2.5–3.0 μm in diameter).

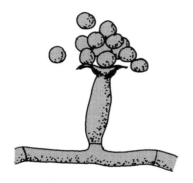
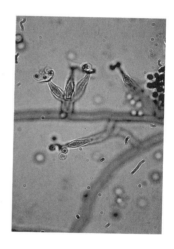

*For more information, see*
 *Kwon-Chung and Bennett, 1992, pp.658–661*
 *Rippon, 1988, pp. 307–311*

---

*Note that *Phialophora repens* and *Phialophora parasitica* also are occasional agents of phaeohyphomycosis. These two species form phialides which typically have inconspicuous, unflared collarettes.

**PATHOGENICITY:**   Causes chromoblastomycosis most commonly in Australia, Venezuela, and South Africa (for description of disease, see p. 121).

**RATE OF GROWTH:**   Slow; mature within 21 days.

**COLONY MORPHOLOGY:**   Dark surface, flat with slightly raised center, covered with velvety dull gray, gray green, or purplish brown short napped mycelium. Reverse is black.

**MICROSCOPIC MORPHOLOGY:**   Hyphae are septate and dark with lateral and terminal conidiophores of various sizes. Conidiation is of the *Cladosporium* type only, i.e., conidiophores produce long, branching chains of brown, smooth-walled, oval, somewhat pointed conidia that are easily dispersed with handling. The conidia typically have dark scars of attachment (i.e., hila). For differentiation from *Xylohypha* spp. and other species of *Cladosporium*, see Table 6.3 (p. 129).

In tissue, the organism appears as large (5–12 µm in diameter), dark, round, septate cells.

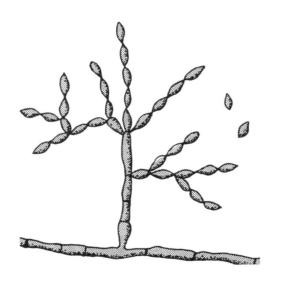
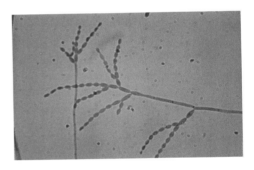

*For further information, see*
  *Kwon-Chung and Bennett, 1992, pp. 350–351*
  *McGinnis, 1980, pp. 198–203*
  *Rippon, 1988, pp. 291, 295*

**TABLE 6.3** Characteristics of *Cladosporium* and *Xylohypha* spp.[a]

| Organism | Distinct conidiophores | "Shield cells" | Shape of conidia | Distinct hila on conidia | Conidial chain length | Conidial chain branching | Maximum growth temp (°C) | Gelatin hydrolysis | Growth with 15% NaCl | Pathogenicity |
|---|---|---|---|---|---|---|---|---|---|---|
| *Cladosporium* spp. | + | + | Oval | + | Short | Frequent | <37 (v)[b] | + (v)[c] | + | Nonpathogenic |
| *Cladosporium carrionii* | ± | ± | Oval | + | Medium | Moderate | 35–37 | − | − | Causes chromoblastomycosis |
| *Xylohypha bantiana* | − | − | Oval | − | Long | Sparse | 42–43 | − | − | Causes cerebral phaeohyphomycosis |
| *Xylohypha emmonsii* | − | − | Bent | − | Medium | Sparse | 37 | − | | Rare cause of subcutaneous phaeohyphomycosis |

[a] Reprinted by permission of the publisher from Larone, 1989. Copyright by Elsevier Science Inc. Abbreviations: +, positive; −, negative; ±, sometimes difficult to distinguish; V, variable.
[b] 29% grow at 40°C.
[c] 86% positive.

**PATHOGENICITY:**   Nonpathogenic; commonly considered a saprophytic contaminant.

**RATE OF GROWTH:**   Moderately rapid, mature within 7 days at 25°C. Most strains do not grow at 37°C, but some do.

**COLONY MORPHOLOGY:**   Surface is greenish brown or black with grayish velvety nap, becoming heaped and slightly folded. Reverse is black.

**MICROSCOPIC MORPHOLOGY:**   Hyphae are septate and dark; conidiophores are dark and branched, vary in length, and usually produce two or more conidial chains. Conidia (3–6 × 4–12 µm) are brown, oval, and usually smooth; they form branching treelike chains and are easily dislodged, showing dark spots (hila) at the point where they were attached to the conidiophore or other conidia. The cells bearing the conidial chains are large and sometimes septate, resemble shields, and may be mistaken for macroconidia when seen alone.

See Table 6.3 (p. 129) for differentiation from pathogenic species of *Clado-sporium.*

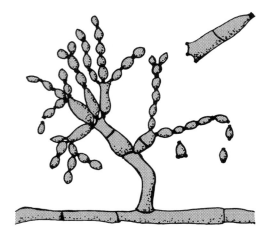
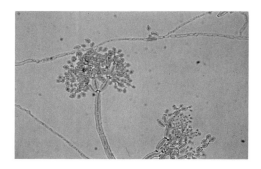

For further information, see
   Barron, 1977, pp. 128–130
   Kwon-Chung and Bennett, 1992, pp. 801–802
   McGinnis, 1980, pp. 198–201, 203
   Rippon, 1988, pp. 771, 773

## *Xylohypha bantiana* (previously known as *Cladosporium bantianum* and *Cladosporium trichoides*)*

**PATHOGENICITY:** The organism has a predilection for the central nervous system and consequently causes cerebral phaeohyphomycosis. Infection might be contracted through inhalation; extreme care and a biological safety cabinet must be used when handling this organism. Slide cultures should NOT be made.

**RATE OF GROWTH:** Slow; mature within 15 days.

**COLONY MORPHOLOGY:** Surface is olive-gray to brown or black and velvety. Reverse is black.

**MICROSCOPIC MORPHOLOGY:** Brown septate hyphae with conidiophores that are similar to the vegetative hyphae; long, sparsely branched wavy chains of smooth oval conidia; the conidia do not display dark scars of attachment. For differentiation from similar organisms, see Table 6.3 (p. 129).

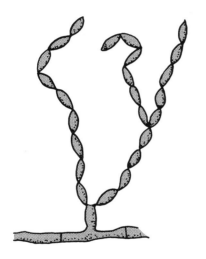

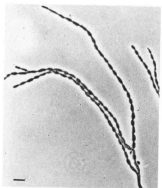

From Michael McGinnis, *Manual of Clinical Microbiology,* 4th ed.

*For further information, see*
  *Kwon-Chung and Bennett, 1992, pp. 642–645*
  *Rippon, 1988, p. 309*

---

*Some mycologists consider *C. bantianum* and *C. trichoides* separate and legitimate species and reject reclassification into the genus *Xylohypha*.

## *Pseudallescheria boydii* (sexual state); *Scedosporium apiospermum* (asexual state)*

**PATHOGENICITY:**   Causes mycetoma (see p. 121 for description of disease). The infection occurs most often in the feet or hands but may occur on any exposed parts of the body. This organism can form pulmonary fungus balls and can also infect the bones, brain, eyes, lungs, sinuses, meninges, and other body sites; it is now clearly recognized as a medically important opportunistic fungus.

**RATE OF GROWTH:**   Moderately rapid; mature in 7 days. The sexual stage (*P. boydii*) is inhibited by cycloheximide; the asexual stage (*S. apiospermum*) is not inhibited.

**COLONY MORPHOLOGY:**   Surface has a spreading, white, cottony aerial mycelium which later turns gray or brown. Reverse is at first white but usually becomes gray or black.

**MICROSCOPIC MORPHOLOGY:**   Hyphae are septate (2–4 μm in diameter), with simple long or short conidiophores bearing conidia singly or in small groups (may resemble mold phase of *Blastomyces dermatitidis*, p. 96). The conidia (4–7 × 5–12 μm) are unicellular and oval, with the larger end toward the apex, and appear cut off at the base (i.e., truncate); they become dark with age. The *Graphium* type of asexual conidiation (p. 146) is seen occasionally; it is characterized by long, erect, narrow conidiophores that are cemented together, diverge at the apex, and bear clusters of oval, truncate conidia (2–3 × 5–7 μm). In the sexual stage, large, brown cleistothecia (50–250 μm in diameter) are formed and release elliptical ascospores when ruptured. The sexual stage may sometimes be induced by culturing on cornmeal agar or potato dextrose agar; the cleistothecia are most likely to form in the center of the colony.

---

*The sexual-stage name has priority over the asexual-stage name. The designation *P. boydii* should therefore be used if the sexual stage is demonstrated; if only the asexual stage is seen, the organism should be called *S. apiospermum.*

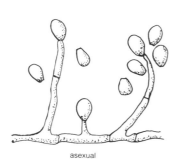

asexual

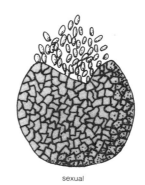

sexual

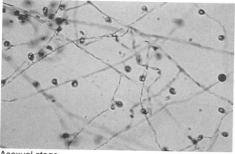

Asexual stage.

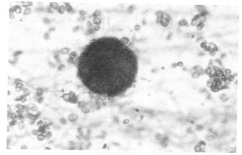

Sexual stage.

*For further information, see*
Kwon-Chung and Bennett, 1992, pp. 577, 678–794
McGinnis, 1980, pp. 172–173, 227–228, 268–271, 505–508
Rippon, 1988, pp. 105, 651–676
Wentworth, 1988, pp. 106–113, 117

**PATHOGENICITY:** Causes invasive infection which is often characterized by arthritis or osteomyelitis. Localized and disseminated infections occur in a variety of sites. Both immunocompromised and immunocompetent patients have presented with infections due to this organism. Asymptomatic colonization has also been reported. The isolates are often resistant to antifungal agents.

**RATE OF GROWTH:** Rapid; mature within 5 days. Growth is inhibited by cycloheximide.

**COLONY MORPHOLOGY:** Young colony is cottony or moist (yeasty) and light gray to black. Mature colony becomes dark grey to black and may develop white mycelial tufts with age. Reverse is gray to black.

**MICROSCOPIC MORPHOLOGY:** Hyphae are septate, with unbranched conidiogenous cells (annellides) having a swollen base and elongated "neck"; conidia form small clusters at the apex. Conidia (2–5 × 3–13 µm) are olive to brown, one celled, smooth, and ovoid with a slightly narrowed, truncated (cut off) base. There is no known sexual state.

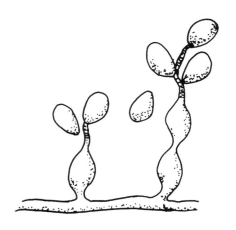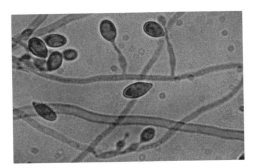

For further information, see
Kwon-Chung and Bennett, 1992, pp. 678–694
Rippon, 1988, pp. 675–676

**PATHOGENICITY:**  *D. constricta* var. *gallopava* has caused subcutaneous and disseminated infections in immunocompromised patients with underlying diseases. The organism is known to have a predilection for the central nervous system and to cause encephalitis in turkeys, chickens, and other birds.

**RATE OF GROWTH:**  Rapid; mature within 5 days.

**COLONY MORPHOLOGY:**  Surface is woolly and dark olive-gray, reddish brown, or gray-black. Reverse is dark; a deep red pigment usually diffuses into the medium.

**MICROSCOPIC MORPHOLOGY:**  Hyphae are septate, with conidiophores that are hyaline, erect, and sometimes knobby or bent at the point of conidial formation. Conidia (average, 3.2 × 9.0 µm) form on threadlike denticles; they are brownish, two celled, and oval to tear shaped and typically have a marked constriction at the central septum. Young conidia may be round and single celled. See Table 6.4 (p. 138) for differentiation of varieties.

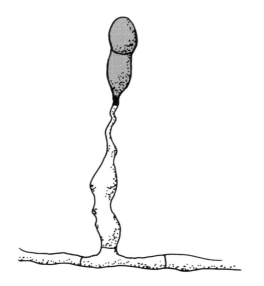

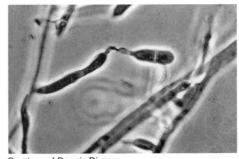

Courtesy of Dennis Dixon.

*For more information, see*
   *Kwon-Chung and Bennett, 1992, pp. 667–668*
   *Dixon and Salkin, 1986*

**PATHOGENICITY:**   Causes mycetoma and phaeohyphomycosis; for description of diseases, see p. 121.

**RATE OF GROWTH:**   Slow; mature within 14 days when incubated at 25–30°C. Grows slower or not at all at 37°C.

**COLONY MORPHOLOGY:**   Surface is at first brownish black or greenish black and skinlike; it then becomes covered with short, velvety, grayish hyphae. Reverse is black.

**MICROSCOPIC MORPHOLOGY:**   Young culture consists of many yeastlike budding cells. Eventually septate hyphae form with numerous conidiogenous cells (annellides) that are slender, tubular, sometimes branched, and characteristically tapered to a narrow, elongated tip. The conidia (1–3 × 2–5 µm) are oval and gather in clusters at the end and sides of the conidiophore and at points along the hyphae. Conidia formation is often best exhibited on cornmeal agar or potato dextrose agar. See Table 6.5 (p. 138) for differentiation from similar organisms.

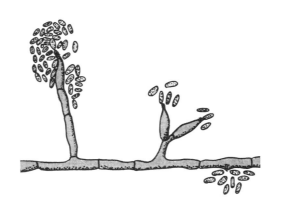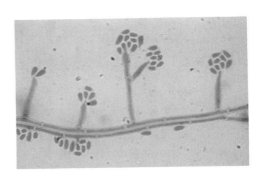

For further information, see
    Kwon-Chung and Bennett, 1992, pp. 575–577, 646–653
    McGinnis, 1980, pp. 211–213, 505–508, 511
    Rippon, 1988, pp. 108–109, 308–309
    Wentworth, 1988, pp. 127–142
For information on other species of Exophiala, see
    Dixon and Polak-Wyss, 1991

**PATHOGENICITY:**   Causes phaeohyphomycosis (for description of disease, see p. 121). The organism appears to have a predilection for the central nervous system; it has been involved in infections of the brain and eye as well as cutaneous and subcutaneous tissue.

**RATE OF GROWTH:**   Slow; mature and filamentous within 25 days (yeastlike in 10 days).

**COLONY MORPHOLOGY:**   At first the colony is black, moist, shiny, and yeastlike. After 3 or 4 weeks or upon repeated subculture, olive-gray aerial hyphae develop at the periphery and sometimes near the center of the colony. Reverse is dark.

**MICROSCOPIC MORPHOLOGY:**   Young cultures are composed of dark (may originally be hyaline), oval to round, budding, yeastlike cells. These cells eventually produce dark, septate hyphae and flask-shaped to cylindric phialides that lack a flared lip. Round to oval, single-celled, pale brown conidia (2–4 × 2.5–6 µm) accumulate at the apex of the phialide and down the sides of the conidiophore. Conidia may also be produced at projections along the hyphae; annellides of the *Exophiala* type have been observed in some isolates. Production of conidia is often sparse. See Table 6.5 (p. 138) for differentiation from similar organisms.

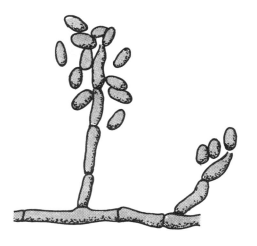
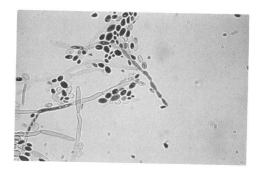

For further information, see
  Kwon-Chung and Bennett, 1992, pp. 647–650
  McGinnis, 1980, pp. 300, 304, 311, 511
  Rippon, 1988, pp. 305–307
  Wentworth, 1988, pp. 141–142, 146–147

**TABLE 6.4**  Differentiation of the varieties of *Dactylaria constricta*[a]

| Organism | Growth with cycloheximide[b] | Gelatinase ≤7 days | Growth at 37–45°C | Pathogenic for humans and birds |
|---|---|---|---|---|
| *D. constricta* var. gallopava | 0 | 0[c] | +[d] | + |
| *D. constricta* var. constricta | + | + | 0 | 0 |

[a] Some mycologists consider the varieties *gallopava* and *constricta* to be separate species, while others place them in the genera *Ochroconis* and *Scolecobasidium.* Abbreviations: 0, negative; +, positive.
   [b] Mycosel agar (BBL, Cockeysville, Md.).
   [c] Delayed positive; ≥21 days.
   [d] Grows more rapidly at 37–45°C than at 30°C.

**TABLE 6.5**  Characteristics of some of the "black yeasts"[a]

| Organism | Decomposition of: | | Growth in 15% NaCl | $KNO_3$ assimilation | Maximum growth temp (°C) |
|---|---|---|---|---|---|
| | Casein (% positive) | Tyrosine (% positive) | | | |
| *Exophiala jeanselmei* | 0 | + (78) | 0 | + | ≤37 |
| *Wangiella dermatitidis* | 0 | + (83) | 0 | 0 | 42 |
| *Phaeoannellomyces werneckii* | + (78) | 0 (22) | + | + | Varying reports |

[a] Reprinted by permission of the publisher from Larone, 1989. Copyright by Elsevier Science Inc. Abbreviations: +, positive; 0, negative.

## Phaeoannellomyces werneckii (*Exophiala werneckii*)

**PATHOGENICITY:** Etiologic agent of tinea nigra, a superficial asymptomatic fungal infection of the skin, usually on the palm of the hands and occasionally on other parts of the body. The lesions are flat, smooth, and not scaly and appear as irregularly shaped brown to black spots resembling silver nitrate stains.

**RATE OF GROWTH:** Develops slowly; mature within 21 days.

**COLONY MORPHOLOGY:** Surface is at first light colored, moist, shiny, and yeastlike but soon becomes olive black. Later grayish-green hyphae form at periphery, and the center loses its shine and becomes olive colored due to thin layer of mycelium. Reverse is black.

**MICROSCOPIC MORPHOLOGY:** The very early phase consists mainly of pale or dark brown yeastlike cells, some having a central septum. These cells (2–5 × 5–10 μm) are actually annellides; they are round at one end while tapered and elongated with striations at the other end where conidia are formed. With age, dark, closely septated, thick-walled hyphae may develop. The one- or two-celled annelloconidia may form and accumulate at annellidic points along the hyphae. Each conidium can function as an annellide and produce new conidia. For characteristics differentiating *Phaeoannellomyces werneckii* from *Wangiella dermatitidis* and *Exophiala jeanselmei*, see Table 6.5 (p. 138).

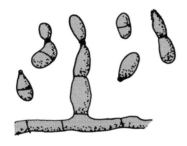
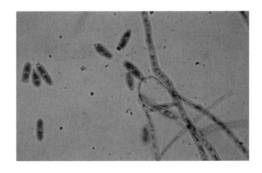

For further information, see
    Kwon-Chung and Bennett, 1992, pp. 191–197
    McGinnis, 1980, pp. 211–213, 215
    Rippon, 1988, pp. 159–163
    Wentworth, 1988, pp. 34–40

**PATHOGENICITY:**   Causes mycetoma (for description of disease, see p. 121).

**RATE OF GROWTH:**   Moderate at 37°C; mature in 10 days. Grows much more slowly at 25° C.

**COLONY MORPHOLOGY:**   Varies greatly; may be smooth or folded and glabrous or powdery and ranges in color from white to yellowish brown. There is usually a brown diffusible pigment in the agar. Reverse is dark brown.

**MICROSCOPIC MORPHOLOGY:**   On Sabouraud dextrose agar, forms only septate hyphae (1–6 μm) with numerous chlamydoconidia-like enlarged cells. On cornmeal agar, some strains produce phialides that bear round or oval conidia at their tips. May form large, black masses of modified hyphae (sclerotia) in old cultures.

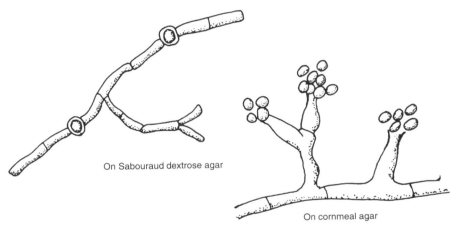

On Sabouraud dextrose agar

On cornmeal agar

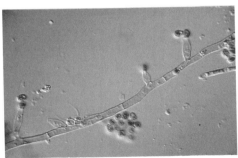

On cornmeal agar. Courtesy of Arvind Padhye.

*For further information, see*
  *Kwon-Chung and Bennett, 1992, pp. 574–579*
  *McGinnis, 1980, pp. 232–234, 236–237, 505–508*
  *Rippon, 1988, pp. 103–107*
  *Wentworth, 1988, pp. 106–114, 117*

**PATHOGENICITY:** Causes mycetoma (for description of disease, see p. 121).

**RATE OF GROWTH:** Moderately slow at 25–30°C; mature in 12 days. Does not grow well, if at all, at 37°C.

**COLONY MORPHOLOGY:** Surface is somewhat folded in the center with radial grooves toward the periphery. Very short, tan or gray aerial hyphae cover a dark gray or olive-brown mycelial mat. Reverse is dark, may form diffusible pigment, but not as commonly as in *M. mycetomatis*.

**MICROSCOPIC MORPHOLOGY:** Hyphae are septate, mostly wide (3–5 μm), branched, and dark. These hyphae sometimes appear to be made up of chains of rounded cells, suggesting a budding process. Thinner (1–3 μm), cylindrical, branched hyphae are also present. Conidia are not commonly formed. Some strains may produce pycnidia; chlamydoconidia are occasionally produced.

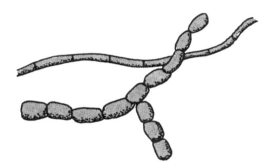 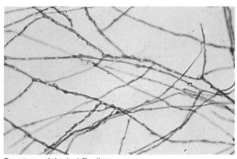

Courtesy of Arvind Padhye.

*For further information, see*
  *Kwon-Chung and Bennett, 1992, pp. 574–575, 579*
  *Rippon, 1988, pp. 104–107*
  *Wentworth, 1988, pp. 106–114, 116–117*

**PATHOGENICITY:** Causes black piedra, a fungal infection of the hairs of the scalp; seen most commonly in the tropics. It is characterized by the formation of small, stony hard, dark nodules along the hair shafts. White piedra is caused by *Trichosporon beigelii* (p. 88).

**RATE OF GROWTH:** Slow; mature in 21 days.

**COLONY MORPHOLOGY:** Colonies are small, adherent, compact, somewhat raised, and dark greenish brown to black and may be glabrous or covered with very short aerial hyphae. Reddish brown diffusible pigment may form. Reverse is black.

**MICROSCOPIC MORPHOLOGY:** Hyphae are closely septate, dark, and thick walled and vary in diameter, with many intercalary chlamydoconidium-like cells. Asci may be produced in culture. The walls of the asci readily dissolve, releasing single-celled, curved, tapering ascospores with whiplike extensions.

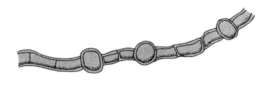

*For further information, see*
  *Kwon-Chung and Bennett, 1992, pp. 183–190*
  *Rippon, 1988, pp. 163–168*
  *Wentworth, 1988, pp. 39–43*

**PATHOGENICITY:**   Commonly considered a contaminant. It has been implicated as an agent of phaeohyphomycosis.

**RATE OF GROWTH:**   Moderately rapid; mature within 7 days.

**COLONY MORPHOLOGY:**   Colony is at first white, but at maturity it is black, shiny, and leathery, with a grayish fringe. Reverse is black.

**MICROSCOPIC MORPHOLOGY:**   Young colonies consist of unicellular, budding, yeastlike cells. Two types of hyphae develop: (i) hyaline, delicate, and thin walled, producing conidia directly from the walls at certain fertile points, and (ii) thick walled, dark, and closely septated, with some cells forming short tubes that produce conidia. Conidia are hyaline and oval (4–6 × 8–12 μm), and continue to multiply by budding. May be confused with *Phaeoannellomyces werneckii* (p. 139) or *Wangiella dermatitidis* (p. 137), but can be distinguished by careful examination of growth rate and microscopic morphology.

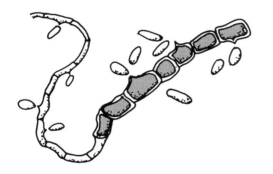 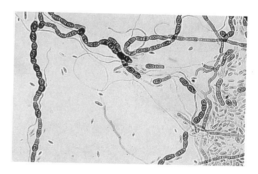

For further information, see
  Barron, 1977, pp. 95–97
  Kwon-Chung and Bennett, 1992, pp. 664–665, 799, 800
  McGinnis, 1980, pp. 186, 191
  Rippon, 1988, pp. 313, 772, 775

---

*Hormonema* sp. is very similar to *A. pullulans*, but it produces conidia in a successive, chainlike fashion from each fertile point; the conidia of *A. pullulans* are produced in synchrony (i.e., simultaneously from separate fertile points).

**PATHOGENICITY:**   Commonly considered a contaminant.

**RATE OF GROWTH:**   Rapid; mature within 5 days.

**COLONY MORPHOLOGY:**   Surface is at first white and then gray or brown, sometimes with blackish spots; woolly. Reverse is usually dark.

**MICROSCOPIC MORPHOLOGY:**   Wide, septate hyphae with dark, septate, long conidiophores that branch only at the apex. The branches have swollen tips that bear round to oval, colorless to pale brown conidia on short denticles. Conidia also form at points along the conidiophore.

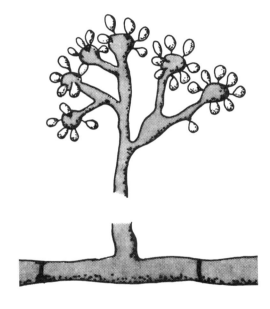

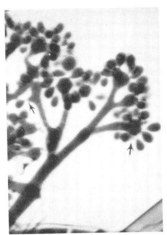

From Rippon, 1988.

*For further information, see*
   *Barron, 1977, pp. 105–106*
   *McGinnis, 1980, pp. 192–193, 195*
   *Rippon, 1988, pp. 760, 761*

## Stachybotrys spp.

**PATHOGENICITY:** Commonly considered a contaminant. *Stachybotrys alternans* produces a potent toxin that is lethal to animals eating contaminated forage. Inhalation or percutaneous absorption has caused mild symptoms in humans.

**RATE OF GROWTH:** Rapid; mature within 4 days.

**COLONY MORPHOLOGY:** Surface is at first white, becoming black with age; cottony, spreading. Reverse is at first light and then dark.

**MICROSCOPIC MORPHOLOGY:** Hyphae are septate and colorless to dark. Conidiophores are simple or branched, may become pigmented and rough with age, and bear clusters of 3–10 phialides. The phialides are colorless or pigmented, nonseptate, and cylindric, with a swollen upper portion. Conidia are dark, oval (average, 4.5 × 9 μm), single celled, and smooth or rough walled and usually form in clusters.

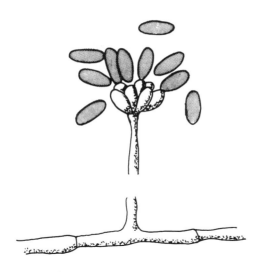 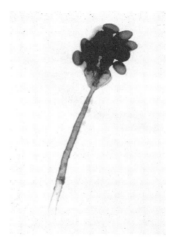

*For further information, see*
  *Barron, 1977, pp. 286–287*
  *Kwon-Chung and Bennett, 1992, pp. 811, 813*
  *McGinnis, 1980, pp. 282–283*
  *Rippon, 1988, pp. 776, 777*

**PATHOGENICITY:**  May be found as a contaminant, but is also an asexual form of *Pseudallescheria boydii* (p. 132).

**RATE OF GROWTH:**  Moderately rapid; mature within 7 days.

**COLONY MORPHOLOGY:**  Surface gray, cottony. Reverse is at first light, turning dark.

**MICROSCOPIC MORPHOLOGY:**  Hyphae are septate, with simple, long, dark conidiophores that are cemented together forming "synnemata." At the apex of each synnema is a cluster of oval, colorless, single-celled conidia (2–3 × 5–7 μm). Delicate rhizoid-like structures appear at the base of the synnema.

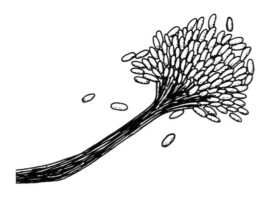 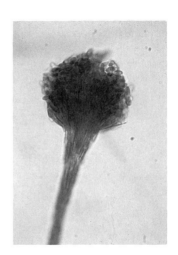

For further information, see
  Barron, 1977, pp. 185–188
  McGinnis, 1980, pp. 227–229

**PATHOGENICITY:**   Known as agents of opportunistic infections of the cornea and sinuses; may cause mycetoma and phaeohyphomycosis at various sites. They are also encountered as contaminants.

**RATE OF GROWTH:**   Rapid; mature within 5 days.

**COLONY MORPHOLOGY:**   Colony is dark olive green to brown or black with a pinkish gray, woolly surface. Reverse is dark.

**MICROSCOPIC MORPHOLOGY:**   Hyphae are septate and dark. Conidiophores are simple or branched and bent or knobby (sympodial geniculate growth) at points of conidium formation. Conidia are large (8–14 × 21–35 μm), usually contain four cells, and may appear curved due to swelling of a central cell. Conidia differ from those of *Bipolaris* spp. (p. 148) by having a central cell that is darker than the end cells, a thinner cell wall, narrower septations between cells, and a distinct curve that develops with age.

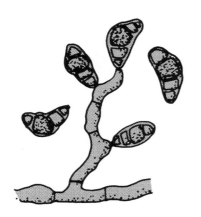 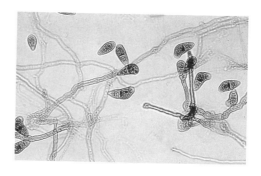

*For further information, see*
  *Barron, 1977, pp. 137–138*
  *Kwon-Chung and Bennett, 1992, pp. 665–666, 802*
  *McGinnis, 1980, pp. 203–204*
  *Rippon, 1988, pp. 311–312, 767*

## *Bipolaris* spp.*

**PATHOGENICITY:**  Occasionally infect a variety of sites including the eye, bones, aorta, sinuses, lung, brain, and skin. Also known to be contaminants in clinical specimens.

**RATE OF GROWTH:**  Rapid; mature within 5 days.

**COLONY MORPHOLOGY:**  Surface is at first grayish brown, becoming black with a matted center and raised grayish periphery. Reverse is black.

**MICROSCOPIC MORPHOLOGY:**  Dark septate hyphae. Conidiophores elongate and bend at the point where each conidium is formed (sympodial geniculate growth); this produces a knobby zigzag appearance. The conidia are brown, thick walled, and oblong to cylindric (6–12 × 16–35 µm) and have three to five septations and a slightly protruding hilum. See Table 6.6 (p. 150) for characteristics that distinguish it from similar organisms.

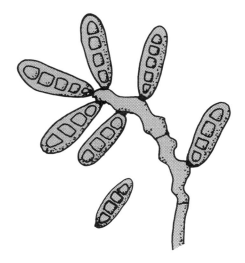
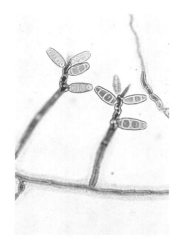

For further information, see
  Kwon-Chung and Bennett, 1992, pp. 653–657, 799–800
  McGinnis et al., 1986
  Rippon, 1988, pp. 316–317

---

*In the past, most isolates of *Bipolaris* sp. were mistakenly called *Drechslera* sp.

**PATHOGENICITY:** Causes phaeohyphomycosis (see p. 121 for description of disease), most commonly in nasal sinuses, skin, and subcutaneous tissue.

**RATE OF GROWTH:** Rapid; mature within 5 days.

**COLONY MORPHOLOGY:** Surface is dark gray to black, cottony. Reverse is black.

**MICROSCOPIC MORPHOLOGY:** Dark septate hyphae. Conidiophores elongate and bend (sympodial geniculate growth) at the point where each conidium is formed; this produces a knobby, zigzag appearance. The conidia are brown, long (average, 14 × 80 µm or greater), fusiform, and thick walled and usually have 7 to 11 septa. The hilum (scar of attachment) on each conidium is seen as a dark, conspicuous, square protrusion. The most commonly encountered species, *E. rostratum*, displays a distinctive dark septum at each end of the mature conidium. See Table 6.6 (p. 150) for differentiation from similar organisms.

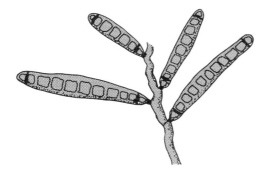 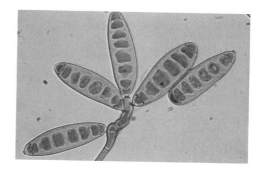

For further information, see
  Kwon-Chung and Bennett, 1992, p. 657
  McGinnis et al., 1986

**TABLE 6.6** Characteristics of *Bipolaris*, *Drechslera*, and *Exserohilum* spp.[a]

| Genus | Reported as pathogen | Conidiation | Conidia Avg. size (μm) | No. of septa | Hilum | Origin | Germ tubes[b] Orientation from basal cell | Illustration |
|---|---|---|---|---|---|---|---|---|
| *Bipolaris* | + | Profuse | 8 × 26 | 3–5 | Protrudes slightly | One or both end cells; adjacent to hilum | Along axis of conidium | |
| *Drechslera* | 0 | Poor | 16 × 65 | 3–5 | Does not protrude | Intermediate and end cells; not adjacent to hilum | Perpendicular to conidial axis | |
| *Exserohilum* | + | Profuse | 14 × 90 or greater | 5–12 | Protrudes strongly | One or both end cells; adjacent to hilum; often other cells | Along axis of conidium | |

[a] Reprinted by permission of the publisher from Larone, 1989. Copyright by Elsevier Science Inc.
[b] See p. 222 for instructions on performance of the germ tube test for these organisms.

**PATHOGENICITY:** Commonly considered a contaminant. Not known to cause infection.

**RATE OF GROWTH:** Rapid; mature within 5 days.

**COLONY MORPHOLOGY:** Surface is dark gray to black, cottony. Reverse is black.

**MICROSCOPIC MORPHOLOGY:** Hyphae are septate. Conidiophores are brown, determinate (i.e., not elongating at the point of conidium formation), slightly curved, unbranched, and often in clusters. Conidia form along the sides of the conidiophores, frequently in whorls. Conidia are large (approximately 9 × 40 μm), dark, and club shaped, with the broader end toward the conidiophore, and usually contain six or more cells.

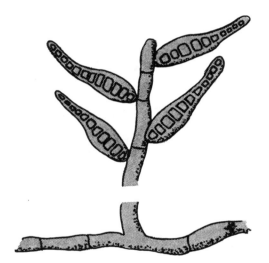
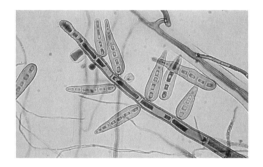

*For further information, see*
  *Barron, 1977, pp. 199–202*
  *McGinnis, 1980, pp. 228–229, 231–232*
  *Rippon, 1988, p. 769*

## *Alternaria* sp.

**PATHOGENICITY:** Commonly considered a saprophytic contaminant but occasionally causes phaeohyphomycosis.

**RATE OF GROWTH:** Rapid; mature within 5 days.

**COLONY MORPHOLOGY:** Surface is at first grayish white and woolly and later becomes greenish black or brown with a light border. May eventually become covered by short, grayish, aerial hyphae. Reverse is black.

**MICROSCOPIC MORPHOLOGY:** Hyphae are septate and dark. Conidiophores are septate and of variable length and sometimes have a zigzag appearance. Conidia are large (7–10 × 23–34 μm) and brown, have both transverse and longitudinal septations, sometimes produce germ tubes, and are found singly or in chains; they are usually rather round at the end nearest the conidiophore, while narrowing at the apex, producing a clublike shape.

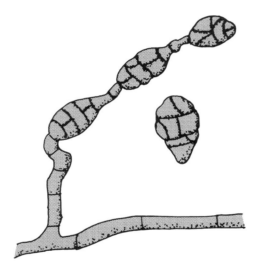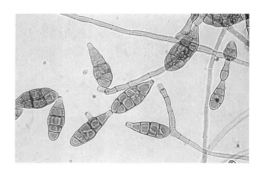

*For further information, see*
  *Barron, 1977, pp. 88–89*
  *Kwon-Chung and Bennett, 1992, pp. 630–631, 662–663*
  *McGinnis, 1980, pp. 181–182*
  *Rippon, 1988, pp. 312–313, 769–770*

**PATHOGENICITY:**   Commonly considered a contaminant; very rarely involved in phaeohyphomycosis.

**RATE OF GROWTH:**   Rapid; mature within 5 days.

**COLONY MORPHOLOGY:**   Surface is dark brown to black, cottony. Reverse is black.

**MICROSCOPIC MORPHOLOGY:**   Septate hyphae, light to dark brown. Conidiophores are simple or branched and bent at points of conidial production, giving a zigzag appearance. Conidia are brown to black, smooth or rough, and round to oval (9–12 × 10–15 µm), with transverse and longitudinal septations.

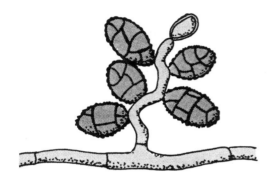
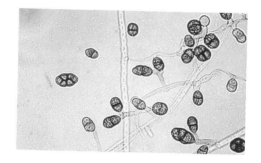

*For further information, see*
*Barron, 1977, pp. 315–317*
*Kwon-Chung and Bennett, 1992, pp. 807–809*
*McGinnis, 1980, pp. 296, 309*
*Rippon, 1988, pp. 769, 771*

## *Stemphylium* sp.

**PATHOGENICITY:**   Commonly considered a contaminant.

**RATE OF GROWTH:**   Rapid; mature within 5 days.

**COLONY MORPHOLOGY:**   Surface is brown to black, cottony. Reverse is black.

**MICROSCOPIC MORPHOLOGY:**   Septate hyphae, light to dark brown. Conidiophores are simple or occasionally branched, with a dark, swollen terminus bearing individual conidia; the conidiophore develops a nodular or knobby appearance as it ages and produces more conidia. Conidia (12–20 × 15–30 µm) are dark, smooth or rough, and round or oval and have transverse and longitudinal septations, often with marked constriction at the central septum.

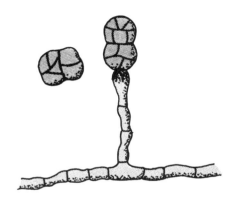 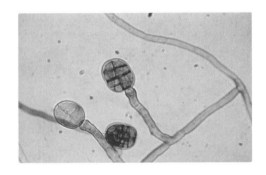

For further information, see
Barron, 1977, pp. 291–292
Kwon-Chung and Bennett, 1992, pp. 811–813
McGinnis, 1980, pp. 283–284
Rippon, 1988, pp. 769, 770

## *Pithomyces* sp.

**PATHOGENICITY:**   Commonly considered a contaminant, but very occasionally has been implicated as an etiologic agent in immunocompromised hosts. Causes facial eczema in sheep.

**RATE OF GROWTH:**   Rapid; mature within 5 days.

**COLONY MORPHOLOGY:**   Surface is light to dark brownish black, cottony. Reverse is dark.

**MICROSCOPIC MORPHOLOGY:**   Septate hyphae, pale or light brown. Conidiophores are short, simple, and peglike. Conidia are single, oval (10–20 × 20–30 μm), yellow to dark brown, and usually rough, with transverse and longitudinal septations.

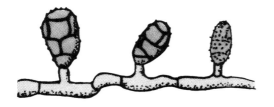
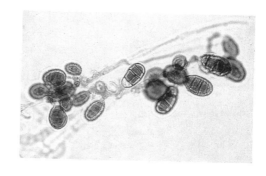

*For further information, see*
*Barron, 1977, pp. 259–260*
*Kwon-Chung and Bennett, 1992, pp. 811, 813*
*Rippon, 1988, pp. 771–772*

**PATHOGENICITY:**   Commonly known as a contaminant.

**RATE OF GROWTH:**   Moderately rapid; mature within 7 days.

**COLONY MORPHOLOGY:**   Colonies are irregularly cottony and usually yellow to orange at first, becoming brown to black with age. Reverse is sometimes red. A diffusible pigment may color the medium yellow, orange, red, or brown.

**MICROSCOPIC MORPHOLOGY:**   Clusters of short conidiophores form on hyphae by repeated branching to form a dense mass from which conidia arise. Young conidia are round to pear shaped, pale, smooth, and nonseptate. Mature conidia (15–30 µm in diameter) are almost round, multiseptate both longitudinally and transversely, dark brown or black, and often rough and warty.

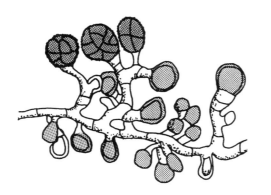 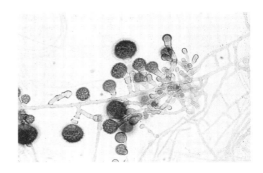

*For further information, see*
  *Barron, 1977, pp. 163–164*
  *Kwon-Chung and Bennett, 1992, pp. 809, 810*
  *McGinnis, 1980, p. 209*
  *Rippon, 1988, pp. 761, 764*

# *Nigrospora* sp.

**PATHOGENICITY:**  Commonly considered a contaminant; not known to be pathogenic.

**RATE OF GROWTH:**  Rapid; mature within 4 days.

**COLONY MORPHOLOGY:**  Compact, woolly; at first white, then gray. With age, black areas of conidiation appear. Reverse is black.

**MICROSCOPIC MORPHOLOGY:**  Hyphae are septate with short conidiophores that swell and then taper at point of conidia formation. The conidia are large, black, and almost round, slightly flattened (approximately 10–14 μm in diameter).

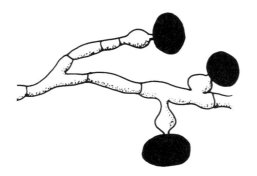 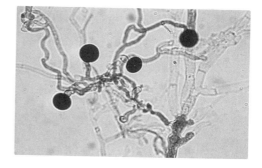

For further information, see
  Barron, 1977, pp. 235–237
  McGinnis, 1980, pp. 241–242, 251
  Rippon, 1988, pp. 771, 774

**PATHOGENICITY:**   Commonly considered a contaminant; occasionally implicated in systemic and cutaneous phaeohyphomycosis.

**RATE OF GROWTH:**   Rapid; mature within 5 days.

**COLONY MORPHOLOGY:**   Surface is cottony, spreading, usually white, becoming tannish gray or grayish olive with age. Reverse is usually orange-tan tinted with red but may be brown to black.

**MICROSCOPIC MORPHOLOGY:**   Hyphae are septate with large (100–150 × 110–225 µm), round, oval, or flask-shaped perithecia (best seen on potato dextrose agar) that are olive to brown and fragile and have wavy and/or straight filamentous appendages. Asci are stalked and club shaped, contain four to eight spores, and usually dissolve soon after release from the ostiole (opening) of the perithecium. Ascospores, readily observed, are oval or lemon shaped, single celled, and usually olive brown but may occur in a variety of sizes, shapes, and colors.

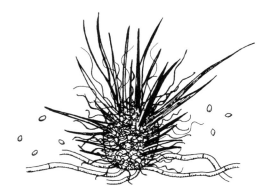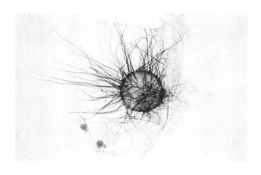

*For further information, see*
  *Kwon-Chung and Bennett, 1992, pp. 666–667, 800–801*
  *McGinnis, 1980, pp. 165–166*
  *Rippon, 1988, pp. 764–765*

**PATHOGENICITY:**   Commonly considered a contaminant. Occasional agent of phaeohyphomycosis.

**RATE OF GROWTH:**   Rapid; mature within 5 days.

**COLONY MORPHOLOGY:**   Colony is powdery or velvety, spreading, and grayish brown. Reverse is black. There is a reddish to brown diffusible pigment in some species.

**MICROSCOPIC MORPHOLOGY:**   Septate hyphae; large (70–100 µm in diameter) asexual fruiting bodies (pycnidia). The pycnidia are dark and round or flask shaped and have openings (ostioles). The conidia, formed on conidiophores inside the pycnidia, are rather oval, one celled, and hyaline.

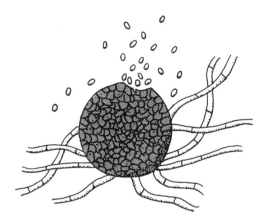 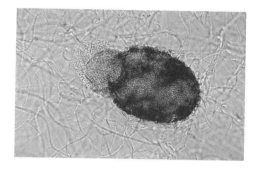

*For further information, see*
   *Kwon-Chung and Bennett, 1992, p. 805*
   *McGinnis, 1980, pp. 178–179*
   *Rippon, 1988, pp. 764, 766*

# Dermatophytes

Dermatophytes are filamentous fungi that are able to digest and obtain nutrients from keratin (a relatively insoluble protein; the primary component of skin, hair, and nails). When the organism grows on the host, living tissue is not usually invaded; the organism simply colonizes the keratinized outermost layer of the skin. The "disease" known as tinea or ringworm is the result of the host reaction to the enzymes released by the fungus during its digestive process. Dermatophytes are the only fungi that have evolved a dependency on human or animal infection for the survival of the species. It is therefore not surprising that these fungi are among the most common infectious agents of humans.

This group is composed of three genera that can generally be differentiated by their formation of conidia:

*Microsporum*:—Macroconidia numerous; thick walled, rough.
   —Microconidia usually present.
   (*M. audouinii* is an exception; it seldom forms conidia)
*Trichophyton*:—Macroconidia rare; thin walled, smooth.
   —Microconidia numerous.
   (Some species do not produce conidia)
*Epidermophyton*:—Macroconidia numerous; thin and thick walled, smooth.
   —Microconidia are not formed.

*For further information, see*
   *Kane et al., in press*
   *Murray et al., 1995, Manual of Clinical Microbiology, 6th ed., chapter 64*

**PATHOGENICITY:**   Formerly caused epidemics of ringworm of the scalp in children. Also known to infect skin on other parts of the body. Very rarely infects adults.

**RATE OF GROWTH:**   Moderate; mature in 7 to 10 days.

**COLONY MORPHOLOGY:**   Surface is flat, downy to silky, and grayish or tannish white. Reverse is light salmon with reddish brown center (pigment is best seen on potato dextrose agar).

**MICROSCOPIC MORPHOLOGY:**   Hyphae are septate with terminal chlamydoconidia that are often pointed on the end. Pectinate (comblike) hyphae are commonly seen. This species is usually almost devoid of conidia but sometimes forms poorly shaped, abortive macroconidia or occasionally microconidia that are identical to those occurring in other species of *Microsporum*.

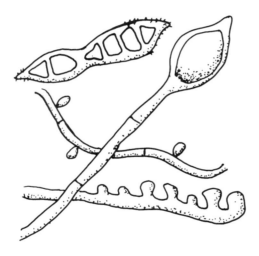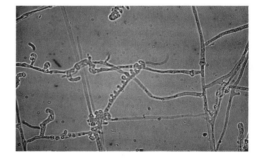

*For further information, see*
  *Kwon-Chung and Bennett, 1992, pp.135–136*
  *Rebell and Taplin, 1970, pp. 16–18*
  *Rippon, 1988, p. 241*
  *Wentworth, 1988, pp. 45–51*

**PATHOGENICITY:** Causes infections of scalp and skin; it is most prevalent in children. Has occasionally been reported as a cause of nail infections. Most infections in humans are acquired from infected dogs or cats.

**RATE OF GROWTH:** Moderate; mature within 6–10 days.

**COLONY MORPHOLOGY:** Surface is whitish, coarsely fluffy, with yellow pigment at periphery and closely spaced radial grooves. Reverse is deep yellow and turns brownish yellow with age.

**MICROSCOPIC MORPHOLOGY:** Hyphae are septate with numerous macroconidia which are long (10–25 × 35–110 μm), spindle shaped, rough, and thick walled and characteristically taper to knoblike ends. The rough surface of the macrconconidia is seen especially at the knob. Usually more than six compartments are seen in the macroconidia. A few microconidia are sometimes observed; they are club shaped and smooth walled and form along the hyphae.

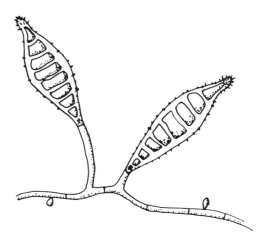
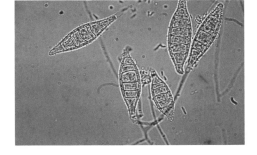

*For further information, see*
 *Kwon-Chung and Bennett, 1992, pp. 136–137*
 *Rebell and Taplin, 1970, pp. 13–14*
 *Rippon, 1988, pp. 241–245*
 *Wentworth, 1988, pp. 47–51, 53*

**PATHOGENICITY:** Occasionally causes ringworm of scalp and other parts of the body.

**RATE OF GROWTH:** Moderate; mature within 6–10 days.

**COLONY MORPHOLOGY:** Surface is fuzzy and flat with raised center; white to buff. Reverse is usually yellow.

**MICROSCOPIC MORPHOLOGY:** Septate hyphae. Macroconidia resemble those of *M. canis* var. *canis* (p. 163) but are very bent and distorted in shape and have fewer compartments; macroconidia are produced best on potato dextrose agar. Club-shaped microconidia are often abundant (an uncommon finding in *M. canis* var. *canis*).

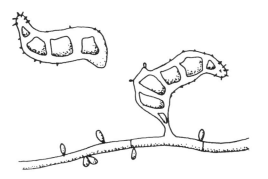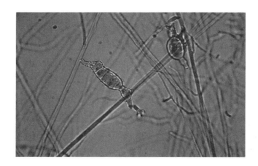

For further information, see
  Kwon-Chung and Bennett, 1992, pp. 136–137
  Rebell and Taplin, 1970, p. 15
  Rippon, 1988, pp. 241–245

**PATHOGENICITY:**  Occasionally involved in infections in humans; it is not known to infect hair in vivo.

**RATE OF GROWTH:**  Moderate; mature within 7 days.

**COLONY MORPHOLOGY:**  Surface is coarse, powdery; yellowish or dark tannish central area surrounded by thin, downy, white peripheral zone. Under the aerial mycelium is a characteristic deep grape-red pigment. Reverse is deep purplish red.

**MICROSCOPIC MORPHOLOGY:**  Hyphae are septate and branched. Macroconidia are oval (10–15 × 30–50 µm), thick walled, and rough, with approximately five to eight cells. Thick walls serve to distinguish this species from reddish isolates of *M. gypseum.* Club-shaped microconidia are usually abundant.

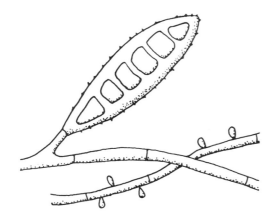 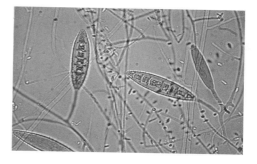

*For further information, see*
  *Kwon-Chung and Bennett, 1992, pp. 142–143*
  *Rebell and Taplin, 1970, p. 29*
  *Rippon, 1988, p. 249*

**PATHOGENICITY:**  Infects the scalp and skin on various parts of the body; infections are more common in lower animals than in humans.

**RATE OF GROWTH:**  Moderately rapid; mature within 6 days.

**COLONY MORPHOLOGY:**  Surface is flat and spreading and powdery to granular, developing an irregularly fringed border; it is buff at first, then tan to cinnamon brown. Colony often develops a sterile white hyphal border or cottony white center. Reverse may be yellow, orange tan, brownish red, or purplish red in spots.

**MICROSCOPIC MORPHOLOGY:**  Septate hyphae. Macroconidia (8–16 × 22–60 µm) appear in enormous numbers and are symmetric, rough, and relatively thin walled with no more than six compartments. The ends are rounded, not pointed as in *M. canis*. Microconidia, club shaped, are usually present along the hyphae.

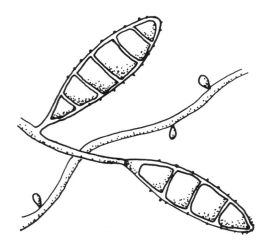 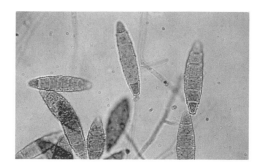

For further information, see
   Kwon-Chung and Bennett, 1992, pp. 138–139
   Rebell and Taplin, 1970, pp. 23–25
   Rippon, 1988, pp. 244–246

**PATHOGENICITY:**   Rare cause of ringworm of the scalp and other parts of the human body; more often seen as cause of ringworm in chickens or other fowl.

**RATE OF GROWTH:**   Moderate; mature in 6–10 days.

**COLONY MORPHOLOGY:**   Surface is slightly fluffy or satiny and white, becoming pinkish with age. Reverse has a red pigment that diffuses into the medium.

**MICROSCOPIC MORPHOLOGY:**   Hyphae are septate. Macroconidia (6–8 × 15–50 µm) have walls that are relatively thin and usually smooth but sometimes slightly rough at the tip; they contain 4–10 cells, are blunt tipped, and are often distinctively curved with a tapering base. Microconidia are usually abundant.

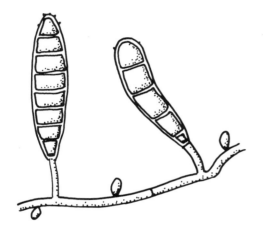 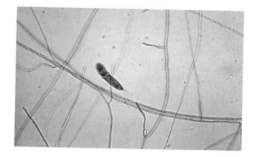

For further information, see
   Kwon-Chung and Bennett, 1992, p. 138
   Rebell and Taplin, 1970, p. 21
   Rippon, 1988, p. 247

**PATHOGENICITY:**   A rare cause of ringworm in humans; more common in pigs.

**RATE OF GROWTH:**   Moderate; mature within 7 days.

**COLONY MORPHOLOGY:**   Surface is at first white and then dark beige, spread thin and powdery. Reverse is initially orange and later reddish brown.

**MICROSCOPIC MORPHOLOGY:**   Septate hyphae; macroconidia (4–8 × 12–18 µm) are rough, fairly thin walled (as in *M. gypseum*), and egg shaped with truncate base, having one to three cells (usually two). Microconidia, club shaped and smooth walled, may also be present.

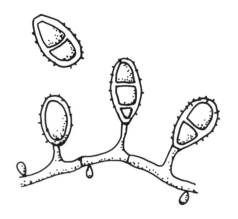 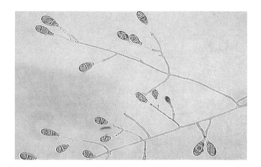

For further information, see
  Kwon-Chung and Bennett, 1992, p. 140
  Rebell and Taplin, 1970, p. 26
  Rippon, 1988, pp. 246–247

**PATHOGENICITY:**   Rare cause of ringworm in humans and lower animals.

**RATE OF GROWTH:**   Moderate; mature within 7 days.

**COLONY MORPHOLOGY:**   Surface is powdery or fluffy; cream, pink, or tan in color. Reverse is colorless or yellow to orange tan.

**MICROSCOPIC MORPHOLOGY:**   Hyphae are septate; macroconidia are long (10–12 × 58–62 μm), tapered, moderately thick walled, and usually rough and spiny surfaced, with seven or more cells. The macroconidia are in abundance singly, laterally, or terminally. Microconidia are also present. Care must be taken not to confuse it with *Trichophyton ajelloi* (p. 182).

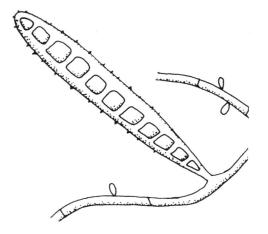 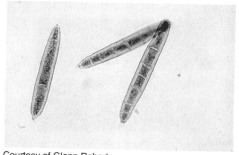

Courtesy of Glenn Roberts.

*For further information, see*
*  Kwon-Chung and Bennett, 1992, p. 141*
*  Rebell and Taplin, 1970, p. 30*
*  Rippon, 1988, p. 249*

**PATHOGENICITY:** Primarily causes ringworm of the scalp (tinea capitis) in children. Also known to infect the skin and nails.

**RATE OF GROWTH:** Slow; mature in 12–20 days.

**COLONY MORPHOLOGY:** Surface is usually yellow to rusty orange, smooth, waxy, heaped; may be flatter and develop a white velvety fuzz. Reverse is cream to brownish. On repeated subculture, organism often loses its pigment.

**MICROSCOPIC MORPHOLOGY:** Hyphae are septate; some are characteristically long and straight with prominent cross walls; these are called "bamboo" hyphae. Other hyphae are irregularly branched, clubbed, and fragmented and may have intercalary chlamydoconidium-like cells. Macroconidia, rarely produced, resemble those of *M. canis* (p. 163) and *M. cookei* (p. 165).

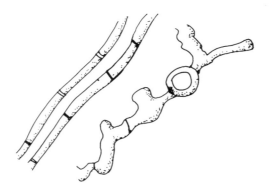
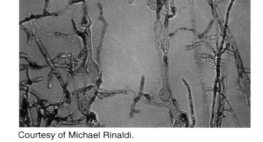

Courtesy of Michael Rinaldi.

For further information, see
Kwon-Chung and Bennett, 1992, pp. 137–138
Rebell and Taplin, 1970, p. 19
Rippon, 1988, p. 245

**PATHOGENICITY:** Invades all parts of the body surface, including hair and nails. It is a common cause of athlete's foot.

**RATE OF GROWTH:** Moderate; mature in 7–10 days.

**COLONY MORPHOLOGY:** Varies greatly; surface may be buff and powdery or white and downy. May become pinkish or yellowish. Powdery form exhibits concentric and radial folds. Colonies rapidly develop a dense fluff with little or no conidiation. Reverse is usually brownish tan but may be colorless, yellow, or red.

**MICROSCOPIC MORPHOLOGY:** Septate hyphae. Macroconidia (4–8 × 20–50 μm) are sometimes, but not always, present; they are cigar shaped and thin walled, have narrow attachment to hyphae, contain one to six cells, and are more readily found in young cultures 5–10 days old. The microconidia in powdery cultures are very round and clustered on branched conidiophores or, in fluffy strains, are smaller, fewer in number, tear shaped, and more easily confused with those of *Trichophyton rubrum* (p. 173). Coiled spiral hyphae are often seen. Nodular bodies are seen in some strains.

See Table 6.7 (p. 172) to differentiate from similar species of *Trichophyton*.

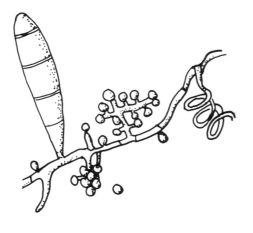
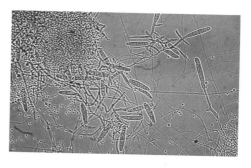

*For further information, see*
  *Kwon-Chung and Bennett, 1992, pp. 143–145*
  *Rebell and Taplin, 1970, pp. 40–43*
  *Rippon, 1988, pp. 252–256*

**TABLE 6.7** Differentiation of similar conidia-producing *Trichophyton* spp.[a]

| Organism | Growth on *Trichophyton* agars | | Urease (7 days) | In vitro hair perforation | Red pigment on cornmeal with 1% dextrose | Growth at 37°C | Growth on *Trichophyton* agars[b] | |
|---|---|---|---|---|---|---|---|---|
| | No. 1 (casein base) | No. 4 (casein + thiamine) | | | | | No. 6 (NH$_4$NO$_3$ base) | No. 7 (NH$_4$NO$_3$ + histidine) |
| *T. mentagrophytes* | 4+ | 4+ | + | + | 0 | + | 4+ | 2+ |
| *T. rubrum* | 4+ | 4+ | 0 or W | 0 | + | + | 3+ | 4+ |
| *T. tonsurans* | ± or + | 4+ | + | 0$^v$ | 0 | + | ± | ± |
| *T. terrestre* | 4+ | 4+ | + | + | V | 0 | 2+ | 2+ |
| *T. megninii* | 2+ | 2+ | +$^v$ | 0 | V | + | 0 | 4+ |

[a] Abbreviations: +, positive; 0, negative; W, weak; ±, trace; 4+, maximum growth; V, variable.
[b] As *T. megninii* is the only dermatophyte that requires histidine, *Trichophyton* agar nos. 6 and 7 are used only when it is suspected; the organism is very rare in the Western Hemisphere.

**PATHOGENICITY:**  Infects the skin and nails and only rarely the beard, hair, or scalp. It is presently the most common dermatophyte to infect humans.

**RATE OF GROWTH:**  Slow; mature within 14 days.

**COLONY MORPHOLOGY:**  Surface is granular or fluffy, white to buff. Reverse is deep red or purplish; occasionally it is brown, yellow orange, or even colorless. The pigment production is best seen on cornmeal dextrose agar (p. 241).

**MICROSCOPIC MORPHOLOGY:**  Hyphae are septate, with lateral, tear-shaped microconidia (2–3 × 3–5 µm). Macroconidia (4–6 × 15–30 µm) may be abundant, rare, or absent; when present, they are long, narrow, and thin walled, with parallel sides, and have two to eight cells. Macroconidia may form directly on ends of thick hyphae singly or in groups. Microconidia characteristically form directly on macroconidia. Arthroconidia tend to form from both hyphae and macroconidia. Granular cultures have more macroconidia formation and larger, rounder microconidia than the fluffy form.

See Table 6.7 (p. 172) for differentiation from similar species of *Trichophyton*.

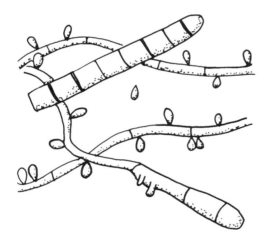 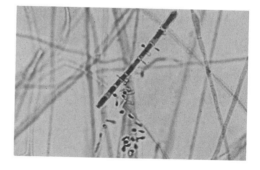

*For further information, see*
  *Kwon-Chung and Bennett, 1992, pp. 145–148*
  *Rebell and Taplin, 1970, pp. 50–51*
  *Rippon, 1988, pp. 255–257*

**PATHOGENICITY:**   The principle etiologic agent of scalp ringworm in the United States; also infects the skin and nails.

**RATE OF GROWTH:**   Moderately slow; mature in 12 days.

**COLONY MORPHOLOGY:**   Highly variable. Surface may be white, grayish, yellow, rose, or brownish. Surface is usually suedelike, with many radial or concentric folds. Reverse is usually reddish brown (pigment may diffuse into the medium); sometimes it is yellow or colorless.

**MICROSCOPIC MORPHOLOGY:**   Hyphae are septate, with many variably shaped microconidia all along the hyphae or on short conidiophores that are perpendicular to the parent hyphae. Microconidia are usually teardrop or club shaped but may be elongate or enlarge to round "balloon" forms. Intercalary and terminal chlamydoconidia are common in older cultures. Macroconidia are rare, irregular in form, and a bit thick walled. May have spiral coils and arthroconidia. This species has a partial requirement for thiamine.

   See Table 6.7 (p. 172) for differentiation from similar species of *Trichophyton*.

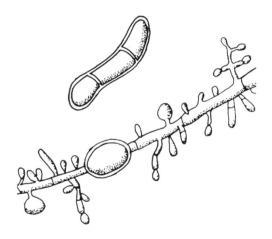
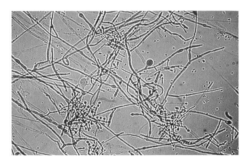

*For further information see*
   *Kwon-Chung and Bennett, 1992, pp. 148–149*
   *Rebell and Taplin, 1970, pp. 52–53*
   *Rippon, 1988, pp. 257–259*

**PATHOGENICITY:**   Primarily causes ringworm of the beard but may also infect the scalp and skin on other parts of the body. Very rarely encountered in the Western Hemisphere.

**RATE OF GROWTH:**   Moderate; mature within 6–10 days.

**COLONY MORPHOLOGY:**   Surface is suede-like, at first white and then pink to violet with widely spaced radial grooves. Reverse is red.

**MICROSCOPIC MORPHOLOGY:**   Hyphae are septate, with teardrop-shaped microconidia. Macroconidia, infrequently produced, are long, narrow (3–6 × 10–35 μm), and pencil shaped. There is a close resemblance to *T. rubrum* (p. 173), but *T. megninii* differs by requiring histidine (in *Trichophyton* agar no. 7) and often giving a positive test for urease within 7 days.

See Table 6.7 (p. 172) for differentiation from similar species of *Trichophyton*.

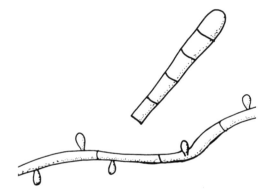
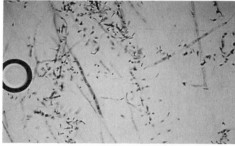

Courtesy of Michael Rinaldi.

*For further information, see*
  *Kwon-Chung and Bennett, 1992, p. 151*
  *Rebell and Taplin, 1970, p. 49*
  *Rippon, 1988, p. 263*

**PATHOGENICITY:**   Not known to cause infection in humans, but may be confused with other *Trichophyton* spp.

**RATE OF GROWTH:**   Moderate; mature within 8 days. It does not grow at 35–37°C.

**COLONY MORPHOLOGY:**   Surface is white to yellow and velvety or granular. Reverse is colorless, yellow, reddish, or brown.

**MICROSCOPIC MORPHOLOGY:**   Hyphae are septate, with characteristic large peg-shaped or club-shaped microconidia that usually exhibit transition forms to rather numerous smooth, thin-walled macroconidia (4–5 × 8–30 µm). The conidia often stain more intensely with lactophenol cotton blue than do the hyphae and are cut off on a relatively broad base.

See Table 6.7 (p. 172) for differentiation from similar species of *Trichophyton*.

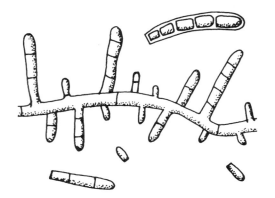 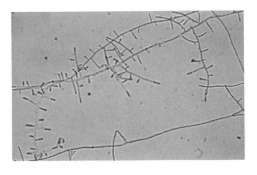

*For further information, see*
  *Rebell and Taplin, 1970, pp. 33–34*

**PATHOGENICITY:**  Primarily infects the scalp and hair and may spread to other parts of the body. It is endemic in Central and West Africa and has been reported in Europe, the United States, and Brazil.

**RATE OF GROWTH:**  Slow; mature within 15 days. Growth is stimulated at 35–37°C. No growth factors are required.

**COLONY MORPHOLOGY:**  Surface is yellow to orange, suede-like, and flat to folded, with a radiating fringe. A purple variant exists. Reverse is similar in color to the surface.

**MICROSCOPIC MORPHOLOGY:**  Septate hyphae break up to form arthroconidia; characteristic branching is at right angles to the parent hypha or backwards (i.e., in a direction opposite to that of the elongating hypha). Teardrop-shaped microconidia may form along the hyphae; no macroconidia are seen.

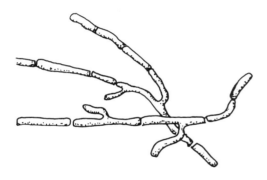
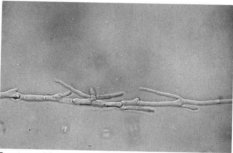

Courtesy of Stanley Rosenthal.

For further information, see
  Kwon-Chung and Bennett, 1992, p. 152
  Rebell and Taplin, 1970, pp. 56–57
  Rippon, 1988, pp. 263–264

**PATHOGENICITY:**   Causes favus, a chronic, scarring scalp infection that results in permanent hair loss; sometimes infects the nails and skin.

**RATE OF GROWTH:**   Slow; mature within 15 days.

**COLONY MORPHOLOGY:**   Colony is whitish, waxy, or slightly downy; heaped or folded; and sometimes yeastlike. Growth is often submerged in the agar. Reverse is colorless or yellowish orange to tan.

**MICROSCOPIC MORPHOLOGY:**   Hyphae are septate and highly irregular and knobby. The subsurface hyphae usually form characteristic antlerlike branching structures commonly called favic chandeliers; they have swollen tips that resemble nailheads. Chlamydoconidia are numerous. Microconidia are rare, and macroconidia are virtually never seen. Initial growth from clinical specimen may resemble yeast both macroscopically and microscopically.
See Table 6.8 (p. 180) for growth pattern on *Trichophyton* agars.

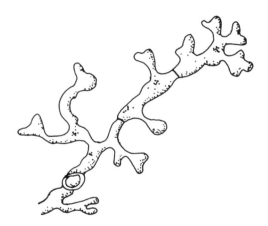
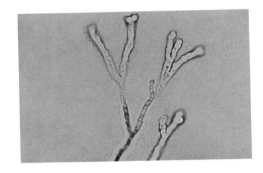

*For further information, see*
  *Kwon-Chung and Bennett, 1992, pp. 149–150*
  *Rebell and Taplin, 1970, pp. 59–60*
  *Rippon, 1988, pp. 260–262*

**PATHOGENICITY:**   Infects scalp, beard, nails, and skin on various parts of the body. Usually contracted from cattle.

**RATE OF GROWTH:**   Slow; mature in 14–21 days. Unlike other dermatophytes, this fungus grows best at 37°C.

**COLONY MORPHOLOGY:**   Usually small, heaped, and buttonlike but sometimes flat. Texture skinlike, waxy, or slightly downy. Usually white, but can be gray or yellow. Reverse varies from nonpigmented to yellow.

**MICROSCOPIC MORPHOLOGY:**   On Sabouraud dextrose agar (SDA) at 37°C, forms hyphae with many chlamydoconidia (often in chains) and some antler-like branches. On enriched media with thiamine, produces many small, delicate, single microconidia and occasional long, thin, irregular macroconidia shaped like string beans or "rats' tails."

See Table 6.8 (p. 180) for growth patterns on *Trichophyton* agars. This species requires thiamine and usually inositol as well.

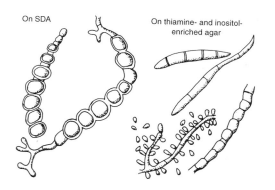

On SDA

On thiamine- and inositol-
enriched agar

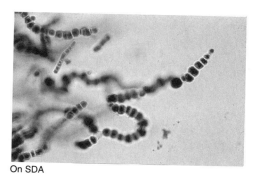

On SDA

*For further information, see*
   *Kwon-Chung and Bennett, 1992, pp. 148–149*
   *Rebell and Taplin, 1970, pp. 47–48*
   *Rippon, 1988, pp. 259–260*

**TABLE 6.8**  Growth patterns of *Trichophyton* species on nutritional test media[a] (p. 250)

| Organism | Percent | Growth on *Trichophyton* agar no. | | | | | | |
|---|---|---|---|---|---|---|---|---|
| | | 1 | 2 | 3 | 4 | 5 | 6 | 7 |
| USUALLY NO CONIDIA ON SABOURAUD AGAR; INCUBATE *TRICHOPHYTON* AGARS AT 37°C | | | | | | | | |
| T. verrucosum | 84 | 0 | ± | 4+ | 0 | | | |
| | 16 | 0 | 0 | 4+ | 4+ | | | |
| T. schoenleini | | 4+ | 4+ | 4+ | 4+ | | | |
| T. concentricum[b] | 50 | 4+ | 4+ | 4+ | 4+ | | | |
| | 50 | 2+ | 2+ | 4+ | 4+ | | | |
| T. violaceum[c] | | ± or 1+ | | | 4+ (in 3 weeks) | | | |
| USUALLY PRODUCES MICROCONIDIA AND SOMETIMES MACROCONIDIA ON SABOURAUD AGAR; INCUBATE *TRICHOPHYTON* AGARS AT ROOM TEMPERATURE | | | | | | | | |
| T. tonsurans | | ± or 1+ | | | 4+ | | | |
| T. rubrum[d] | | 4+ | | | 4+ | | | |
| T. mentagrophytes[d] | | 4+ | | | 4+ | 4+ | | |
| T. equinum[e] | | 0 | | | | 4+ | | |
| T. megninii[f] | | 4+ | | | 2+ | | 0 | 4+ |
| T. terrestre[g] | | 4+ | | | 4+ | | | |

[a]Abbreviations: 1, casein agar base (vitamin free);
2, casein + inositol;
3, casein + inositol and thiamine;
4, casein + thiamine;
5, casein + nicotinic acid;
6, ammonium nitrate agar base;
7, ammonium nitrate + histidine;
0, no growth;
+, growth;
4+, maximum growth.

[b]For more information, see Rebell and Taplin (1970, p. 61).

[c]Usually has distinct pigment on primary isolation.

[d]Differentiation of *T. rubrum* and *T. mentagrophytes* is by morphology, urease test, in vitro hair perforation test, and pigment production on cornmeal dextrose agar. See Table 6.7.

[e]Commonly found in horses; has been confused with *T. mentagrophytes*, but *T. equinum* usually requires nicotinic acid. For more information, see Rebell and Taplin (1970, p. 45).

[f]No other dermatophyte shows this regular requirement for histidine.

[g]Not known to cause infections, but may be confused with some pathogenic species. See Table 6.7.

**PATHOGENICITY:**  Infects the scalp, hair, skin, and nails.

**RATE OF GROWTH:**  Slow; mature in 14–21 days.

**COLONY MORPHOLOGY:**  Original cultures are waxy, wrinkled, heaped, and deep purplish red. Subcultures are more downy, and they decrease in color. Reverse is lavender to purple.

**MICROSCOPIC MORPHOLOGY:**  Hyphae are tangled, branched, irregular, and granular, with intercalary chlamydoconidia. Microconidia and macroconidia are not usually seen on Sabouraud dextrose agar, but a few may form on thiamine-enriched media.

See Table 6.8 (p. 180) for growth pattern on *Trichophyton* agars. This species has a partial requirement for thiamine.

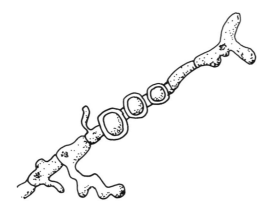

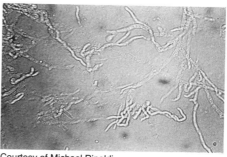

Courtesy of Michael Rinaldi.

*For further information, see*
*Kwon-Chung and Bennett, 1992, pp. 150–151*
*Rebell and Taplin, 1970, p. 54*
*Rippon, 1988, p. 259*

**PATHOGENICITY:**  Has only rarely been reported as a possible cause of infections in humans.

**RATE OF GROWTH:**  Moderate; mature within 7 days.

**COLONY MORPHOLOGY:**  Surface is cream to orange tan, rather powdery, and flat or folded. Reverse may be colorless or have a reddish purple or bluish black pigment that diffuses into the medium.

**MICROSCOPIC MORPHOLOGY:**  Hyphae are septate with many macroconidia that are long (5–10 × 20–65 µm), cigar shaped or cylindric with tapering ends, smooth surfaced, and moderately thick walled and that contain 5 to 12 cells. Microconidia may be abundant in some isolates and sparse to absent in others. Care must be taken not to confuse this organism with *Microsporum vanbreuseghemii* (p. 169) or *Epidermophyton floccosum* (p. 183).

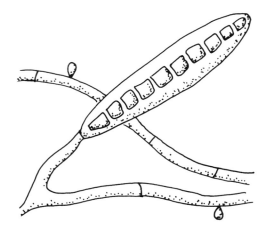

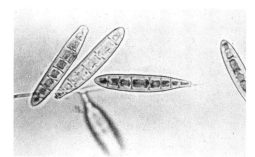

From Weitzman and Kane, *Manual of Clinical Microbiology,* 5th ed.

*For further information, see*
  *Rebell and Taplin, 1970, p. 31*
  *Rippon, 1988, pp. 263–265*

**PATHOGENICITY:**   Produces infection in skin and nails (not hair).

**RATE OF GROWTH:**   Moderate; mature within 10 days.

**COLONY MORPHOLOGY:**   Surface is brownish yellow to olive gray or khaki; it is at first lumpy and sparse and then folded in center and grooved radially, becoming velvety. After several weeks, fluffy white sterile mycelium covers the colony. Reverse is orange to brownish, sometimes with a thin yellow border.

**MICROSCOPIC MORPHOLOGY:**   Septate hyphae; no microconidia. Macroconidia (7–12 × 20–40 µm), seen best in young cultures, are smooth, both thin and slightly thick walled, and club shaped with rounded ends; they contain two to six cells and are found singly or in characteristic clusters. With age, macroconidia often transform into chlamydoconidia.

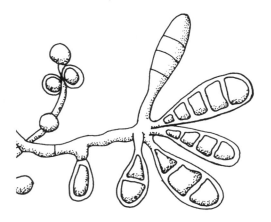 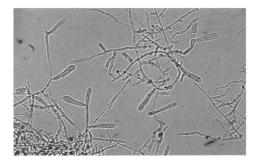

*For further information, see*
  *Kwon-Chung and Bennett, 1992, p. 154*
  *Rebell and Taplin, 1970, p. 62*
  *Rippon, 1988, pp. 266–269*

# ■ Hyaline Hyphomycetes

This section contains the fungi that have not been discussed earlier in this guide. These molds have colorless, septate hyphae and produce conidia that may be colorless or pigmented. Their colony surface is white, gray, tan, yellow, pink, or green; the reverse is white or lightly pigmented. Some of these organisms are known pathogens (e.g., *Coccidioides immitis*), but most of them are opportunistic and cause disease only in the immunocompromised patient.

In the past, all fungi were categorized as pathogens or saprophytes—those days are gone forever. Almost any fungus isolated from a clinical specimen might be an etiologic agent of infection in a predisposed individual. All fungal isolates should be identified; most of those commonly considered saprophytes are identified only to genus level, as it often requires an expert to differentiate the species.

In the medical laboratory, the saprophytic fungi are frequently encountered as contaminants. The source of the organism may be the transport container, the medium, or the laboratory environment, but most often it is the site from which the specimen was taken. Every effort should be made to instruct the clinicians on proper techniques for specimen collection.

Other fungi that are commonly considered saprophytes, contaminants, and/or possible opportunists are described in previous sections of this guide.

*For further information, see*
  *Murray et al., 1995, Manual of Clinical Microbiology, 6th ed., chapters 63 and 67*

**PATHOGENICITY:** Causes coccidioidomycosis, which is a highly infectious disease that may be an acute but benign, self-limiting respiratory disease or a chronic, malignant, sometimes fatal infection involving the skin, bone, joints, lymph nodes, adrenals, and central nervous system. It is endemic in the arid southwestern United States and in dry regions of Mexico, Central America, and South America.

**RATE OF GROWTH:** Moderate; mature within 10 days. Growth occurs in 3–5 days, but production of arthroconidia may take 1–2 weeks.

**COLONY MORPHOLOGY:** There may be great variation in colony morphology. On Sabouraud dextrose agar (SDA) at 25 or 37°C the colony often is at first moist, grayish, and membranous and soon develops a white, cottony aerial mycelium, which becomes gray or tan to brown with age. Reverse is white to gray. Only when grown on special medium at 37–40°C is the spherule, or tissue phase, formed in vitro.

**MICROSCOPIC MORPHOLOGY:** Cultures exhibit coarse, septate, branched hyphae that produce thick-walled, barrel-shaped arthroconidia (2–4 × 3–6 μm) that alternate with empty cells. The walls of the empty cells break and are characteristically present on either end of the freed conidia. Racquet hyphae are present in young colonies. Careful microscopic examination should prevent confusion with *Geotrichum candidum* (p. 89). To confirm the identity of *C. immitis* and differentiate it from the saprophytes that it very closely resembles, it is necessary to perform one of the following tests: (i) specific DNA probe (commercially available), (ii) immunodiffusion test for exoantigen (usually performed by reference laboratories), (iii) cultivation of spherules in special synthetic medium in increased $CO_2$ tension at 37–40°C, or (iv) animal inoculation for in vivo production of spherules.

   In tissues or body fluids, *C. immitis* exists as large, round, thick-walled spherules (10–80 μm in diameter), which contain endospores (2–5 μm in diameter). Immature nonendosporulating cells may resemble nonbudding forms of *Blastomyces dermatitidis*. When cultured on routine media, whether incubated at 25, 30, or 37°C, the organism is filamentous (for that reason, it is not placed with the thermally dimorphic fungi in this guide).

   *Note*: Because the arthroconidia are highly infectious, the cultures must be handled with great care and grown in tubes only, not petri plates. The tubed growth should be wet down with sterile water before handling. A biological safety cabinet must be used. Slide cultures should NOT be made.

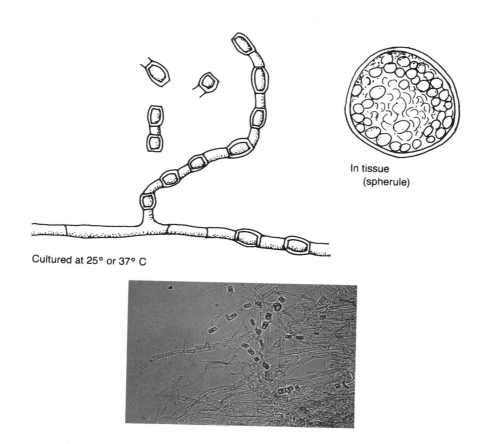

In tissue
(spherule)

Cultured at 25° or 37° C

For further information, see
  Evans and Richardson, 1989, pp. 148–151
  Kwon-Chung and Bennett, 1992, pp. 356–396
  McGinnis, 1980, pp. 201–203, 484–486
  Rippon, 1988, pp. 433–473
  Saubolle and Sutton, 1994

THERMALLY MONOMORPHIC MOLDS    **187**

## *Emmonsia parva (Chrysosporium parvum)**

**PATHOGENICITY:** Causes adiaspiromycosis, a pulmonary disease seen mainly in rodents and occasionally in humans. This mycosis is characterized by the in vivo enlargement, without multiplication, of inhaled conidia. *E. parva* var. *crescens* is the variety most associated with human infection; *E. parva* var. *parva* has very rarely been reported. The mycosis is usually self limited, benign, localized, and relatively asymptomatic; a few fatal cases have occurred.

**RATE OF GROWTH:** Moderate; mature in 7–14 days. For primary isolation, minced lung tissue should be cultured on routine mycology agar at 25°C; the organism will grow in the presence of cycloheximide. *E. parva* has NOT been isolated from sputum or bronchioalveolar lavage fluid.

**COLONY MORPHOLOGY:** Surface is white, occasionally buff to pale brown in the center; some areas may be glabrous while others have tufts of matted mycelia; slight radial grooves may form. Reverse is cream to pale brown.

**MICROSCOPIC MORPHOLOGY:** Hyphae are septate (1–2.5 µm in diameter), sometimes in cemented clumps. Conidiophores are at right angles to the vegetative hyphae and produce single or short chains of conidia that are slightly oval (2–4 × 2.5–4.5 µm) and sometimes rough walled. The conidia may also form directly on short stalks along the sides of the hyphae. At this stage, the morphology is indistinguishable from some *Chrysosporium* spp. (p. 203).

When the hyphae and conidia are incubated at elevated temperatures, the hyphae become distorted and usually disintegrate while the conidia swell to become round thick-walled adiaspores. The adiaspores of *E. parva* var. *crescens* are produced at 37°C, are multinucleate (up to several hundred nuclei), and measure 100 µm or greater in diameter. The adiaspores of *E. parva* var. *parva* are best produced at 40°C, are uninucleate, and range from 10–25 µm in diameter.

At various temperatures and stages of development, *E. parva* may resemble a number of other fungi including *Blastomyces dermatitidis*, *Paracoccidioides brasiliensis*, *Histoplasma capsulatum*, and *Chrysosporium* spp.

*Note*: Isolates may give false-positive results with the *Blastomyces dermatitidis* DNA probe, exoantigen, and direct immunofluorescent antigen tests.

---

*The name to be applied to this organism is presently under consideration.

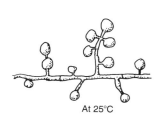

At 25°C

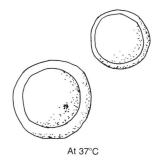

At 37°C

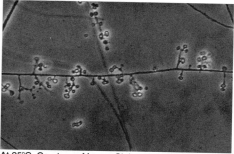

At 25°C. Courtesy of Lynne Sigler.

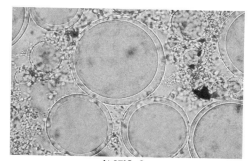

At 37°C. Courtesy of Lynne Sigler.

*For further information, see*
    *Kwon-Chung and Bennett, 1992, pp. 733–739*
    *Rippon, 1988, pp. 718–721*

**TABLE 6.9** Identification of the most common species of *Aspergillus* (see description of genus on p. 192)

| A. fumigatus[a] | A. niger | A. flavus | A. versicolor |
|---|---|---|---|
| **PATHOGENICITY** Most common cause of aspergillosis | Usually considered a contaminant, but also known to cause disease in the debilitated | Usually a contaminant but also known to cause disease; commonly associated with aflatoxins | Usually considered a contaminant, but has been known to cause disease |
| **MACROSCOPIC MORPHOLOGY**[b] Velvety or powdery, at first white, then turning dark greenish to gray. Reverse white to tan | Wooly, at first white to yellow, then turning black. Reverse white to yellow | Velvety, yellow to green or brown. Reverse goldish to red brown | Velvety; at first white, then yellow, orangey, tan, green, or occasionally pinkish. Reverse white; may be yellow, orange, or red |
| **MICROSCOPIC MORPHOLOGY OF CONIDIOPHORES** Short (<300 µm) Smooth | Long Smooth | Variable length Rough, pitted, spiny | Long Smooth |
| **MICROSCOPIC MORPHOLOGY OF PHIALIDES** Uniseriate, usually only on upper two-thirds of vesicle, parallel to axis of conidiophore | Biseriate, cover entire vesicle, form "radiate" head | Uniseriate and biseriate, cover entire vesicle, point out in all directions | Biseriate, loosely radiate, cover most of vesicle (Hülle cells may be present) |

[a] *A. fumigatus* grows well at 45°C or higher.
[b] Classically studied on Czapek-Dox agar; on Sabouraud dextrose agar, most species of *Aspergillus* grow luxuriantly but not always characteristically.

| A. nidulans | A. glaucus group | A. terreus | A. clavatus |
|---|---|---|---|
| **PATHOGENICITY** | | | |
| Usually considered a contaminant, but has been involved in infections | Commonly known as a contaminant, but also known to cause infection under certain conditions | Commonly considered a contaminant, but also known to cause infection | Commonly considered a contaminant |
| **MACROSCOPIC MORPHOLOGY**[b] | | | |
| Velvety; usually green, but buff to yellow where cleistothecia form. Reverse purplish red becoming dark | Feltlike; green with yellow areas; occasionally brown. Reverse yellowish to maroon (grows best with 20% sucrose added to the medium) | Usually velvety, cinnamon brown. Reverse white to brown | Feltlike, blue green. Reverse white, may become brown with age |
| **MICROSCOPIC MORPHOLOGY OF CONIDIOPHORES** | | | |
| Short (<250 μm) Smooth, brown | Variable length Smooth | Short (<250 μm) Smooth | Long Smooth |
| **MICROSCOPIC MORPHOLOGY OF PHIALIDES** | | | |
| Biseriate, short columnar. Cleistothecia usually present with reddish ascospores; Hülle cells often abundant. | Uniseriate, radiate to very loosely columnar, cover entire vesicle (cleistothecia generally present) | Biseriate, compactly columnar (round hyaline cells produced on mycelium submerged in agar) | Uniseriate, closely crowded on huge clavate vesicle (approximately 200 × 40 μm) |

**PATHOGENICITY:** Members of the genus cause a group of diseases known as aspergillosis. The disease may be in the form of invasive infection, colonization, toxicoses, or allergy. Species of *Aspergillus* are opportunistic invaders, infecting various sites in individuals with lowered resistance due to underlying immunocompromising, debilitating disease and/or prolonged treatment with immunosuppressive drugs or antimicrobial agents. *Aspergillus* spp. are widespread in the environment and are commonly found as contaminants in cultures.

**RATE OF GROWTH:** Usually rapid; mature within 3 days; some species are slower growing.

**COLONY MORPHOLOGY:** Surface is at first white and then any shade of yellow, green, brown, or black, depending on species. Texture is velvety or cottony. Reverse is white, goldish, or brown.

**MICROSCOPIC MORPHOLOGY:** Hyphae are septate (2.5–8.0 μm in diameter); an unbranched conidiophore arises from a specialized foot cell. The conidiophore is enlarged at the tip, forming a swollen vesicle. Vesicles are completely or partially covered with flask-shaped phialides (formerly referred to as sterigmata) which may develop directly on the vesicle (uniseriate form) or be supported by a cell known as a metula (biseriate form). The phialides produce chains of mostly round, sometimes rough, conidia (2–5 μm in diameter).

See Table 6.9 (p. 190) for differentiation of species most commonly encountered in the clinical laboratory.

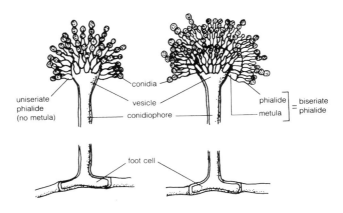

*For further information, see*
  *Evans and Richardson, 1989, pp. 159–163*
  *Kwon-Chung and Bennett, 1992, pp. 201–247*
  *McGinnis, 1980, pp. 182–190, 475–477*
  *Rippon, 1988, pp. 618–650*
  *Wentworth, 1988, pp. 174–183*
*For detailed descriptions and keys to all species of Aspergillus, see*
  *Raper and Fennell, 1973*

**PATHOGENICITY:**   Commonly considered a contaminant, but found in a variety of diseases in which its etiologic significance is uncertain. It has been known to cause keratitis (inflammation of the cornea), external ear, respiratory, and urinary tract infections, and endocarditis after insertion of valve prostheses. Disseminated disease has been reported in a patient with acute leukemia. Some strains produce toxins.

See also *Penicillium marneffei* (p. 100).

**RATE OF GROWTH:**   Rapid; mature within 4 days.

**COLONY MORPHOLOGY:**   Surface at first is white, then becomes very powdery and bluish green with a white border. Some less common species differ in color and texture. Reverse is usually white, but may be red or brown. If the isolate produces a red reverse and diffuse pigment in the agar, *P. marneffei* (p. 100) must be considered and the organism should be tested for thermal dimorphism; this is especially relevant if the patient has recently visited southeast Asia.

**MICROSCOPIC MORPHOLOGY:**   Hyphae are septate (1.5–5 µm in diameter) with branched or unbranched conidiophores that have secondary branches known as metulae. On the metulae, arranged in whorls, are flask-shaped phialides that bear unbranched chains of smooth or rough, round conidia (2.5–5 µm diameter). The entire structure forms the characteristic "penicillus" or "brush" appearance.

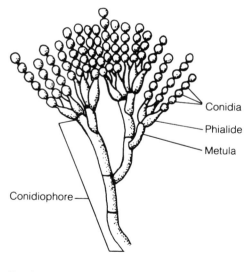

Conidia

Phialide

Metula

Conidiophore

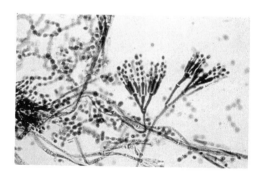

*For further information, see*
*Barron, 1977, pp. 247–248*
*Kwon-Chung and Bennett, 1992, pp. 750–752, 804–805*
*McGinnis, 1980, pp. 251–261*
*Rippon, 1988, pp. 728–730, 754–755*

**PATHOGENICITY:** Usually considered a contaminant, but is increasingly associated with disease, especially keratitis (inflammation of the cornea). It has also been reported to cause endocarditis, sinusitis, nephritis, cutaneous and subcutaneous infections, pulmonary infection, and fungemia.

**RATE OF GROWTH:** Rapid; mature within 3 days.

**COLONY MORPHOLOGY:** Surface is flat and powdery or velvety; usually yellowish brown, it is sometimes lilac or another color. Reverse is off-white to brown.

**MICROSCOPIC MORPHOLOGY:** Resembles *Penicillium* spp. (p. 193), but the phialides of *Paecilomyces* spp. are more elongated and taper into a long, slender tube, giving them the shape of tenpins; they bend away from the axis of the conidiophore and may appear singly along the hyphae. The conidia (approx. 2 × 3.5 µm) are elliptical or oblong and occur in long, unbranched chains.

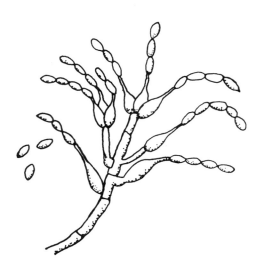 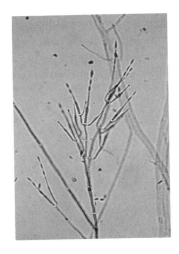

For further information, see
Barron, 1977, pp. 244–246
Kwon-Chung and Bennett, 1992, pp. 747–750, 753, 803–804
McGinnis, 1980, pp. 244, 247–248
Rippon, 1988, pp. 735–736, 756

**PATHOGENICITY:**   Commonly considered a contaminant, but is known to infect the nails (usually toenail) and is rarely associated with infection of soft tissue, bone, and lungs in immunocompromised patients.

**RATE OF GROWTH:**   Rapid; mature within 5 days.

**COLONY MORPHOLOGY:**   Surface is at first white and glabrous and then usually becomes powdery light brown with a light tan periphery. Some rarely encountered species may be very dark. Reverse is tan with brownish center.

**MICROSCOPIC MORPHOLOGY:**   Septate hyphae; *Scopulariopsis* spp. somewhat resemble *Penicillium* spp. (p. 193) but they have shorter and sometimes simpler conidiophores, and the conidia-bearing cells are annellides and may be more cylindric; the conidia are larger (4–9 μm in diameter), often thick walled, round to lemon shaped, and cut off at the base, forming a short neck. The mature conidia are usually very rough and spiny.

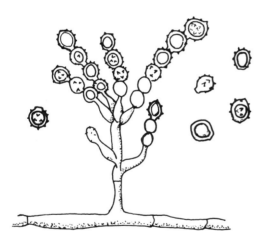
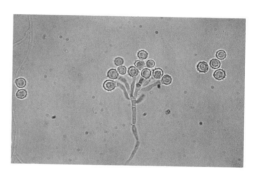

For further information, see
   Barron, 1977, pp. 275–278
   Kwon-Chung and Bennett, 1992, pp. 752–753, 806–807
   McGinnis, 1980, pp. 272–275
   Rippon, 1988, pp. 736, 756, 758

**PATHOGENICITY:**   Commonly known as a contaminant.

**RATE OF GROWTH:**   Rapid; mature within 4 days.

**COLONY MORPHOLOGY:**   Surface is at first white. The center then becomes dark green; some strains may be pinkish. Fluffy growth spreads over plate in one week. Reverse is white.

**MICROSCOPIC MORPHOLOGY:**   The hyphae, conidiophores, and phialides are similar to those of *Penicillium* spp. (p. 193); however, the conidia of *Gliocladium* do not remain in chains but clump together with the conidia of adjacent phialides to form large clusters or balls.

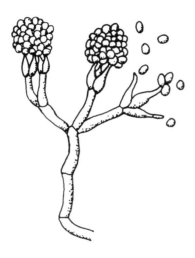
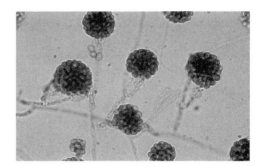

For further information, see
   Barron, 1977, pp. 177–179
   Kwon-Chung and Bennett, 1992, pp. 809–810
   McGinnis, 1980, pp. 224, 226
   Rippon, 1988, pp. 756–757

**PATHOGENICITY:** Commonly considered a contaminant; very occasionally associated with infection in the immunocompromised patient.

**RATE OF GROWTH:** Rapid; mature within 5 days.

**COLONY MORPHOLOGY:** White fluff covers agar in a few days and then becomes more compact and woolly. Green patches are eventually produced due to formation of conidia. Reverse is colorless or light orangey tan to yellow.

**MICROSCOPIC MORPHOLOGY:** Hyphae are septate, conidiophores are short and often branched at wide angles, and phialides are flask shaped and form at wide angles to the conidiophore. Conidia (average, 3 μm in diameter) are round, single celled, and clustered together at the end of each phialide. Clusters are easily disrupted unless microscopic preparations are handled with exceptional care.

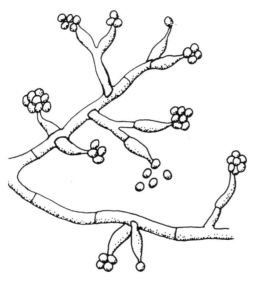
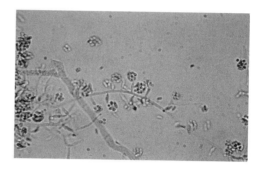

*For further information, see*
  *Barron, 1977, pp. 306–307*
  *Kwon-Chung and Bennett, 1992, pp. 754–755, 812–814*
  *McGinnis, 1980, pp. 288–289*
  *Rippon, 1988, pp. 756, 758*

**PATHOGENICITY:**   Commonly considered a contaminant. Known to be pathogenic in some animals and insects; very rarely involved in infection of humans.

**RATE OF GROWTH:**   Rapid; mature within 4 days.

**COLONY MORPHOLOGY:**   Surface is white to cream, occasionally pinkish; fluffy to powdery. Reverse is white.

**MICROSCOPIC MORPHOLOGY:**   Narrow, delicate, septate hyphae (approximately 1.5 µm in diameter) are seen. Conidia-producing structures are rather flask shaped with a narrow zigzag terminal extension bearing a conidium at each bent point (sympodial geniculate growth). Conidia are small (2–4 µm in diameter), one celled, and round to oval, each forming singly on a tiny denticle. It is best to examine young cultures before dense clusters of conidiogenous cells form, making it difficult to observe the characteristic arrangement of conidia.

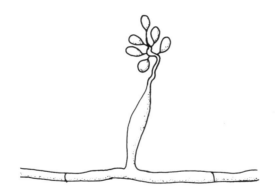 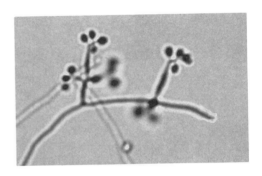

For further information, see
   Barron, 1977, pp. 98–99
   Kwon-Chung and Bennett, 1992, pp. 745, 799–800
   McGinnis, 1980, pp. 186–187, 192–193
   Rippon, 1988, pp. 730–731, 760

**PATHOGENICITY:** Commonly known as a contaminant. Reported as rare agent of keratitis (inflammation of the cornea).

**RATE OF GROWTH:** Rapid; mature within 4 days.

**COLONY MORPHOLOGY:** Surface is at first white and then may become pinkish brown, red, green, or yellow; powdery or velvety in texture; spreading. Reverse is white or rust in color.

**MICROSCOPIC MORPHOLOGY:** Septate hyphae. Conidiophores are simple or branched at several levels and in whorls (i.e., verticillate); phialides are very elongate, having pointed apex, also arranged in whorls. Conidia are oval and single celled, appear singly or in clusters at ends of phialides, and remain in place only if slide preparations are handled with great care.

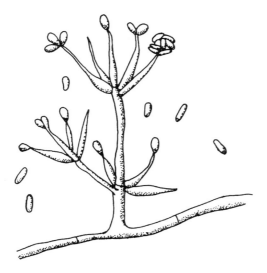
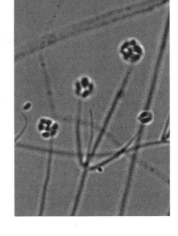

*For further information, see*
  *Barron, 1977, pp. 321–323*
  *McGinnis, 1980, pp. 296, 300, 310*
  *Rippon, 1988, pp. 757, 759*

**PATHOGENICITY:** Etiologic agent of mycetomas, corneal infections, and nail infections. Invasive disease at various body sites has been reported on rare occasion. It is also encountered as a contaminant.

**RATE OF GROWTH:** Rapid; mature within 5 days.

**COLONY MORPHOLOGY:** At first it is compact, folded, and feltlike and then becomes overgrown with loose, white, cottony hyphae. May be white, gray, or rose in color. Reverse is colorless, pale yellow, or pinkish.

**MICROSCOPIC MORPHOLOGY:** Extremely delicate. Hyphae are septate; erect, unbranched, tapering phialides form directly on the fine, narrow hyphae. Conidia are oblong (2–3 × 4–8 μm) and usually one celled but occasionally two celled. The conidia form easily disrupted clusters at the tips of the phialides.

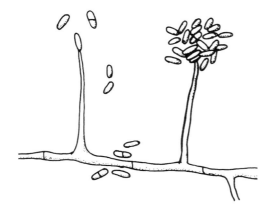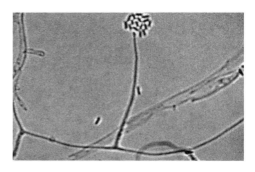

For further information, see
Barron, 1977, pp. 114–116
Kwon-Chung and Bennett, 1992, pp. 573–575, 577, 744–745, 797–798
McGinnis, 1980, pp. 179–181
Rippon, 1988, pp. 109–110, 731–732, 761, 763

**PATHOGENICITY:**  Commonly considered a contaminant, but known to be a relatively frequent agent of mycotic eye infections. It is occasionally involved in mycetoma, sinusitis, skin and nail infections, and disseminated systemic infections in severely debilitated hosts. Disease has also been reported in individuals after ingestion of food prepared from grain that had been overgrown by toxin-producing species.

**RATE OF GROWTH:**  Rapid; mature within 4 days.

**COLONY MORPHOLOGY:**  At first it is white and cottony, but it often quickly develops a pink or violet center with a lighter periphery. Some species remain white or become tan. Reverse is light in color.

**MICROSCOPIC MORPHOLOGY:**  Septate hyphae. There are two types of sporulation: (i) large (3–8 × 11–70 µm), sickle- or canoe-shaped, multiseptate macroconidia produced from phialides on unbranched or branched conidiophores and (ii) long or short, simple conidiophores bearing small (2–4 × 4–8 µm), oval, one- or two-celled conidia singly or in clusters resembling those of *Acremonium* spp. (p. 200).

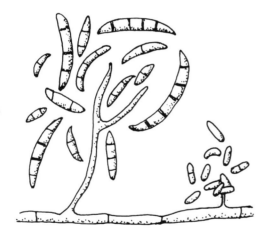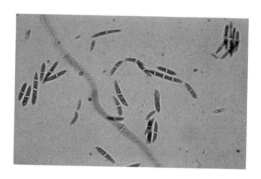

For further information, see
   Barron, 1977, pp. 164–166
   Kwon-Chung and Bennett, 1992, pp. 574–575, 745–752, 802–803
   McGinnis, 1980, pp. 218–220, 223
   Rippon, 1988, pp. 732–735, 757, 759

**PATHOGENICITY:**   Commonly considered a contaminant.

**RATE OF GROWTH:**   Rapid; mature within 4 days.

**COLONY MORPHOLOGY:**   At first it is white and woolly and then becomes pink or peach colored. Reverse is light.

**MICROSCOPIC MORPHOLOGY:**   Septate hyphae. Conidiophores are long, slender, and mostly unbranched. Conidia (8–10 $\times$ 12–18 µm) are smooth, slightly thick walled, two celled, and pear or club shaped, with a well-marked truncate attachment point frequently off to one side, forming a "foot." The conidia are produced in alternating directions and remain side by side in an elongated group.

   The long conidiophores and the smooth walls, attachment points, and arrangement of the conidia serve to distinguish this organism from *Microsporum nanum* (p. 168).

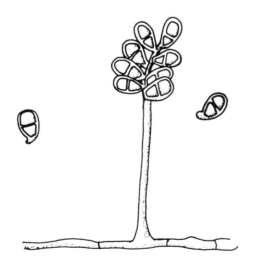
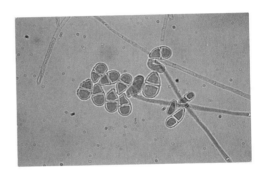

For further information, see
   *Barron, 1977, pp. 309–310*
   *Kwon-Chung and Bennett, 1992, pp. 812, 814*
   *McGinnis, 1980, pp. 293–294, 303, 304*

**PATHOGENICITY:** Commonly considered a contaminant. Rarely reported in association with infections, mainly in toenails.

**RATE OF GROWTH:** Moderately rapid; mature within 6 days.

**COLONY MORPHOLOGY:** Varies greatly. Cottony, powdery, or granular; flat or raised; usually white, yellow, or tan to pale brown, but may be pink, orange, or gray. Reverse is usually white to brown, but may be another color.

**MICROSCOPIC MORPHOLOGY:** Septate hyphae. Conidia are one celled (2–4 × 3–7 µm), ovoid, and smooth or rough walled with a broadly truncate base and a broad basal scar and often carry a remnant of the hyphal wall after detachment from the hypha. Conidia are borne singly or in short chains at tips of conidiophores or branching hyphae, directly on sides of hyphae, on short pedicels, or in intercalary positions.

The morphology resembles that of *Emmonsia parva* (p. 188), but adiaspores do not develop at 37°C; some species will not grow at 37°C. Young conidium formation may mimic that of *Blastomyces dermatitidis* (p. 96).

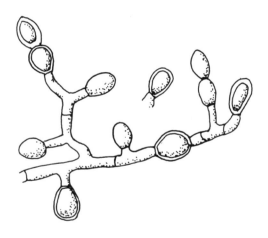 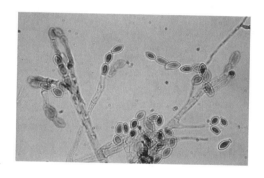

For further information, see
  Barron, 1977, pp. 125–127
  Kwon-Chung and Bennett, 1992, pp. 753–754, 801
  McGinnis, 1980, pp. 197–199
  Rippon, 1988, pp. 760, 763

**PATHOGENICITY:** Commonly considered a contaminant.

**RATE OF GROWTH:** Rapid; mature within 5 days.

**COLONY MORPHOLOGY:** Surface is velvety to granular; at first it is white and then becomes tan, pinkish, yellow, or orange. Reverse is tannish.

**MICROSCOPIC MORPHOLOGY:** Hyphae are broad, lightly pigmented, and septate with bridges known as clamp connections at the septa. Short, simple conidiophores bear conidia which are single celled, ovoid (average, 6 × 10 μm), golden, and cut off sharply at the base and which often retain a portion of attached conidiophore after separation. The conidial walls are fairly thick and may be smooth or rough.

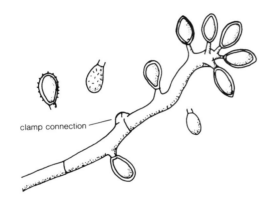

clamp connection

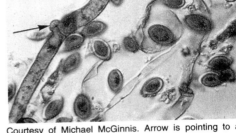

Courtesy of Michael McGinnis. Arrow is pointing to a clamp connection.

*For further information, see*
  *Barron, 1977, pp. 285–286*
  *McGinnis, 1980, pp. 279–281*

**PATHOGENICITY:**   Commonly considered a contaminant.

**RATE OF GROWTH:**   Moderately rapid; mature within 7 days.

**COLONY MORPHOLOGY:**   At 25°C, colonies are at first white and waxy, then become fluffy, and with age often turn yellow. At 37°C there is little or no growth. Reverse is white.

**MICROSCOPIC MORPHOLOGY:**   Hyphae are septate with simple or branched conidiophores. Conidia are large (7–17 µm), round, thick walled, and usually rough and knobby. Differs from *Histoplasma capsulatum* (p. 94) by not forming microconidia, not converting to a yeast at 35–37°C, and not reacting with the DNA probe specific for *H. capsulatum.*

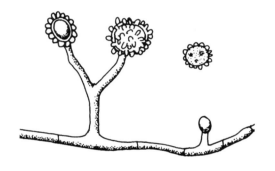 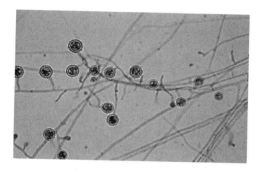

*For further information, see*
   *Barron, 1977, pp. 278–279*
   *Kwon-Chung and Bennett, 1992, p. 493*
   *McGinnis, 1980, pp. 276–278*
   *Rippon, 1988, pp. 760, 762*

**PATHOGENICITY:**   Commonly considered a contaminant; rarely involved in infections of the cornea.

**RATE OF GROWTH:**   Rapid; mature within 3 days.

**COLONY MORPHOLOGY:**   White at first and then salmon colored. Thin fluff rapidly spreads over surface of agar.

**MICROSCOPIC MORPHOLOGY:**   Hyphae are septate; simple conidiophores produce branching chains of oval conidia by continuous budding. The older hyphae break up, forming thick-walled arthroconidia.

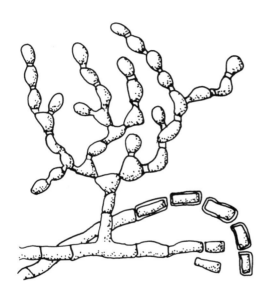

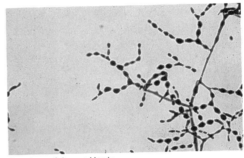

Courtesy of James Harris.

*For further information, see*
  *Barron, 1977, p. 227*
  *McGinnis, 1980, pp. 238–239, 247*

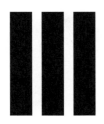

# Laboratory Technique

# Laboratory Procedures

# 7

## Collection and Preparation of Specimens

No matter how experienced the mycologist, isolation and identification of fungi from clinical specimens are not likely to be accomplished unless the specimen is properly collected and sent immediately to the laboratory. All specimens should be transported in sterile containers and processed as soon as possible. If a specific fungus is suspected by the physician, the laboratory should be notified as special media and cultural procedures may be needed, and the information will be helpful for the safety of laboratory personnel.

Consult references (p. 212) if more information on specimen handling is required.

BLOOD. Blood for fungal cultures must be collected aseptically and inoculated into broth or tubes containing sodium polyanethol sulfonate in a final concentration of 0.03–0.05%; the incorporation of saponin to lyse the blood cells is also desirable. Since recovery of fungi increases with the volume of blood tested and since fungal sepsis may be intermittent, at least two blood samples should be separately collected and cultured. Broth bottles should be vented upon receipt in the laboratory.

Special methods and media for fungal blood cultures are now commercially available from a variety of manufacturers. The lysis-centrifugation system (ISO-LATOR, Wampole Laboratories, Cranbury, N.J.) has been shown to detect more fungi in less time than the more conventional methods. It is definitely the method of choice for the detection and isolation of *Histoplasma capsulatum*. The automated blood culture systems (BacT/Alert [Organon Teknika, Durham, N.C.], BACTEC [Becton Dickinson, Sparks, Md.], and ESP [Difco Laboratories, Detroit, Mich.]) are improved by using broth specifically designed for the culturing of fungi. If a manual method is to be used, biphasic blood culture medium consisting of broth with an agar slant (e.g., Septi-Chek; Becton Dickinson, Cockeysville, Md.) is significantly better than broth alone. With all commercial systems, manufacturers' instructions should be followed.

Conventional broth blood cultures may require 20–30 days before becoming positive and should be subcultured at regular intervals regardless of gross appearance.

The membrane filter technique has long been a very successful means of recovering yeasts from blood. For membrane filtration, 8 ml of blood is collected in sodium polyanethol sulfonate (yellow-stoppered Vacutainer tube, Becton Dickinson) and a 0.45-μm-pore-size filter is used. The specimen should be kept no longer than 1 h at 35–37°C before filtering.

BONE MARROW.    Samples of bone marrow should consist of at least 0.5 ml of aspirated marrow. The pediatric ISOLATOR (Wampole Laboratories) is well designed for this small-volume culture. Alternatively, the specimen can be collected in a heparinized syringe and inoculated onto appropriate fungal media at the bedside. Many laboratories use the same bottled broth methods as those used for fungal blood cultures (see above). The specimen should also be smeared and stained with Giemsa or Wright stain for *Histoplasma capsulatum*.

CEREBROSPINAL FLUID (CSF).    CSF should be centrifuged at 2,000 × $g$ for 10 min. The supernatant fluid should not be decanted unless a portion is needed for cryptococcal antigen testing. With a sterile pipette, the sediment is removed and used to inoculate the medium and prepare smears for microscopic examination. Any remaining sediment is resuspended and the medium is reinoculated with fairly large amounts of the whole specimen. If less than 2 ml of specimen is received, it should be inoculated directly onto the media. Filtration of CSF through a 0.45-μm-pore-size membrane filter, followed by culture of the filter, is sometimes the preferred method.

CUTANEOUS SPECIMENS

*Skin.* Specimens of skin are taken from an area previously cleansed with 70% alcohol. The active, peripheral edge of a lesion is scraped with a scalpel or the end of a microscope slide, and the scales are placed in a sterile petri dish.

*Nails.* When nails are suspected of fungal infection, they should be cleansed with an alcohol wipe and then scraped deeply enough to obtain recently invaded nail tissue. The initial scrapings should be discarded, as they are usually contaminated.

*Scalp and Hair.* Invaders of the scalp and hair are best isolated by culturing the basal portion of the infected hair. Infected hairs may be selected by placing the patient under a UV light (Wood's lamp); hairs infected with some dermatophytes fluoresce under UV light. Hairs that are fluorescent, distorted, or fractured should be cultured.

EXUDATES, PUS, AND DRAINAGE.    Specimens of exudates, pus, and drainage should be examined for granules by using a dissecting microscope. If granules are present, the color is noted and then a portion of the specimen is teased apart gently, crushed between two glass slides, and examined microscopically; the remainder is washed several times in sterile distilled water, crushed with a sterile glass rod, and inoculated onto appropriate media (granules may be bacterial and should be plated accordingly). If no granules are present, the specimen is examined microscopically for hyphae and other fungal elements and directly inoculated onto isolation media.

EYE.    Eye cultures for fungi are most successful when the medium is directly inoculated by the ophthalmologist. Corneal scrapings are transferred from a platinum spatula to an agar plate (blood agar plates are the most commonly used) by making a series of C-shaped cuts on the medium. Scraped material should also be smeared on alcohol-cleaned, flamed slides.

FLUIDS.    Fluids (e.g., pleural, peritoneal, or joint fluids) must sometimes be collected with heparin to prevent clotting. The fluid is centrifuged at 2,000 $\times$ $g$ for 10 min; any clotted material should be minced with a sterile scalpel and combined with the concentrated fluid. At least 0.3 ml of inoculum is placed onto each medium. The use of lysis-centrifugation (ISOLATOR, Wampole Laboratories) is a recommended alternative.

SPUTUM.    Sputum should be collected as a first early morning sample after the patient's teeth are brushed and the mouth is well rinsed; 24-h specimens are not satisfactory, as they become easily overgrown with bacteria and saprophytic fungi. Flecks containing pus, blood, or caseous material should be sought and used in culture and smears. Sputum decontaminated for culturing acid-fast bacilli is not acceptable because the sodium hydroxide in the procedure destroys a large number of fungi; concentration methods employing a mucolytic agent without sodium hydroxide may be used, but they have not been shown to increase the recovery rate of fungi from clinical specimens.

STOOL.    Specimens of stool are rarely worth culturing for fungi, as their presence in such a contaminated material is usually without meaning. Growth of a large amount (predominance) of yeast has possible significance, but colonization is very common in both healthy individuals and compromised patients.

TISSUES.    Tissues should be minced with a scalpel or ground with a mortar and pestle or tissue grinder. If necessary, a small amount of sterile saline or broth may be added to facilitate grinding. If infection with a Zygomycete is suspected, the tissue should be minced, not ground or homogenized, as these procedures destroy the hyphae and decrease the viability of the organisms. Direct microscopic examination is best accomplished with thin paraffin sections stained with Gomori methenamine silver. Subcutaneous tissue should be carefully examined for granules; if granules are present, they should be handled as described previously (see section on exudates, pus, and drainage).

URINE.     Urine should be collected in a sterile container as a first morning "midstream" specimen. Upon reaching the laboratory, the urine is centrifuged at 2,000 × $g$ for 10 min, the supernatant is decanted, and approximately 0.5 ml of the sediment is placed on each medium to be used. If quantitation is required, a calibrated loop is used to streak uncentrifuged urine onto a plate of appropriate medium. The interpretation of the colony count is still under dispute. The clinical presentation of the patient must be given prime consideration in the determination of the significance of *Candida* spp. in urine.

*For further information on collection and preparation of specimens, see*
  *Evans and Richardson, 1989, pp. 3–12, 24–45*
  *Isenberg, 1992, pp. 6.1.1–6.1.5, 6.6.1–6.6.5*
  *McGinnis, 1980, pp. 88–99*
  *Murray et al., 1995, Manual of Clinical Microbiology, 6th ed., chapter 59*
  *Wentworth, 1988, pp. 11–32*

## Methods for Direct Microscopic Examination of Specimens

Any specimen submitted for fungus culture can be examined microscopically for fungal elements. This examination is made in addition to, not instead of, a culture. As well as providing the physician with early information regarding the possible need for treatment, it may be helpful in determining the significance of the organism that will later be identified on culture. For a guide to interpreting direct microscopic examinations of clinical specimens, see chapter 1 (p. 9–17).

### POTASSIUM HYDROXIDE (KOH) PREPARATION

Most organic substances that might be confused with fungi when seen through the microscope are converted to an almost clear background in the presence of moderately strong alkaline solutions. The fungi remain unaffected and are therefore rather easily demonstrated. Ink, added to the KOH, stains fungal elements and helps them stand out from the background.

#### Reagent (clearing and staining agent)

1. Make a 10% KOH solution in Parker Super Quink Ink, permanent blue-black (50 ml of ink + 5 g of KOH pellets).
2. Centrifuge KOH-ink solution at 2,500 rpm for 10 min.
3. Pour supernatant into plastic (not glass) sterile tube. Store at room temperature.

**Slide preparation**

1. Place a portion of the specimen on a labeled slide.
2. Add 1 drop of KOH-ink solution to the slide; mix.
3. Put a coverslip over the preparation.
4. Heat gently over flame. *Do not boil*; portions of nails may demand repeated and prolonged heating for the necessary degree of chemical softening so that the material can be pressed out to afford good visibility.
5. The slide must be carefully examined microscopically to detect hyphal segments, spores or conidia, budding yeasts, spherules, or sclerotic bodies. Cotton swabs should not be used in preparing these slides, as the cotton strands may resemble hyphae.

KOH preparations are not permanent; the reagent will eventually destroy the fungi. The addition of a small amount of glycerol to the preparation will preserve it for several days.

## INDIA INK PREPARATION

A drop of India ink is placed on a glass slide and mixed with a loopful of centrifuged (2,000 × *g* for 10 min) spinal fluid sediment or a small amount of isolated yeast. A coverslip is added, and the slide is examined for yeast cells with capsules. Sputum or pus can be cleared with KOH and heat and then mixed with India ink. If the India ink is too dark, it may be diluted with sterile distilled water.

Capsular material is exhibited by the appearance of a clear, well demarcated halo around a yeast cell. When seen in CSF it is suggestive of *Cryptococcus neoformans*, but identification must be confirmed by culture and biochemical testing of the isolate. Other species and other genera also produce capsules. The capsules of cryptococci vary from 2–10 μm or more in width; they tend to be small in specimens from immunodeficient patients. Leukocytes may also appear haloed, but the halo has a fuzzy, irregular appearance at the periphery, and the cell within the halo has a much paler cell wall than does *C. neoformans*.

Cryptococci often lose their ability to produce capsules when grown on artificial media.

The cryptococcal latex antigen test has been proven to be significantly more sensitive than the India ink preparation and is therefore recommended for the initial diagnosis of cryptococcal disease.

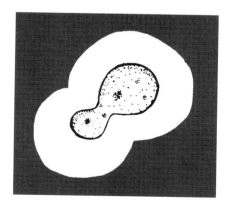

## STAINED PREPARATIONS

1. Calcofluor white (p. 227) is an excellent fluorescent stain for detection of fungi in specimens. It can be combined with KOH (discussed above) if clearing is required. It is a valuable tool and is highly recommended.

2. Gram stain (p. 230) is most useful in the mycology laboratory for examining specimens for the presence of aerobic actinomycetes. It is commonly used in bacteriology laboratories and may demonstrate mycelial elements and yeast cells, but it does not usually allow for the best observation of morphologic features.

3. A modified Kinyoun acid-fast stain (p. 225) is used to detect the partially acid-fast filaments of *Nocardia* spp. The routine Kinyoun method is used to stain ascospores.

4. Wright's stain (commonly performed in hematology laboratories) or Giemsa stain (p. 228) is used for detecting intracellular yeast forms of *Histoplasma capsulatum* in blood and bone marrow.

5. The periodic acid-Schiff (PAS; customarily performed in histology laboratories) and Gomori's methenamine silver (GMS; p. 228) stains are considered the best for demonstrating fungi in tissue.

## Primary Isolation

Specimens to be cultured for fungus must be inoculated onto media that, in combination, will ensure the growth of all fungi that may be clinically significant. Several possible batteries of media can be used, and the ultimate choice often depends on factors such as cost, availability, and personal preference. In any case, the battery should include media with and without antibiotics. Cycloheximide is incorporated in media to inhibit the rapidly growing saprophytic fungi which could overgrow slow growing primary pathogens. It is necessary to use media lacking cycloheximide to grow the organisms that are commonly considered saprophytes or contaminants but can act as opportunistic pathogens; in addition, cycloheximide is known to inhibit the growth of some significant pathogens, e.g., *Cryptococcus neoformans*, *Penicillium marneffei*, *Aspergillus fumigatus*, *Pseudallescheria boydii*, some *Candida* species, and most Zygomycetes. Chloramphenicol and/or gentamicin are commonly employed to inhibit bacterial contamination. It is also generally recommended that an enriched medium be used to ensure the growth of very fastidious thermally dimorphic fungi.

The routine use of the readily available, commercially prepared media listed in Table 7.1 fulfills the requirements for primary culture of clinical specimens.

Whenever possible, and unless otherwise indicated, at least 0.5 ml of specimen should be inoculated onto each agar surface. Media should be slanted in large tubes and optimally left in a horizontal position (on an acid-fast bacilli culture rack) for 24 h after inoculation in order for the inoculum to remain dispersed rather than to accumulate at the bottom of the slant. The tubes can then be stood vertically for subsequent incubation. The screw caps must be kept partially loosened to ensure proper atmospheric conditions. Petri plates provide a larger surface area for isolation of fungi but are more hazardous to handle. If plates are used, they should contain 40 ml of medium and be surrounded by a shrink seal to prevent dehydration; the shrink seal also prevents unintentional opening. Plates should NOT be used if *Coccidioides immitis* is suspected.

**TABLE 7.1** Suggested battery of primary culture media[a]

| Medium | Purpose |
|---|---|
| Sabouraud dextrose agar (SDA) (Emmons modification preferred) | Provides the standard, classic morphology, not necessarily the best growth or sporulation; usually supports growth of aerobic actinomycetes. |
| SDA with cycloheximide and chloramphenicol (Mycobiotic or Mycosel agar) | Inhibits most saprophytic fungi (but also some pathogenic fungi) and most bacteria. |
| Inhibitory mold agar (IMA) | Enriched medium containing chloramphenicol or gentamicin; supports growth of almost all molds and yeasts while inhibiting bacteria. |
| Brain-heart infusion (BHI) agar | Supports the growth of fastidious thermally dimorphic fungi. Recovery is somewhat improved with the incorporation of 5–10% sheep blood, but organisms must be subcultured to a blood-free medium to induce conidiation. Culture with BHI agar may be deleted when specimens are not likely to contain fastidious fungi (e.g., specimens of hair, nail, skin for dermatophytes, mouth, throat, nose, vagina, cervix, urine, or stool). |

[a]When just a small amount of cerebrospinal fluid or bone marrow is available, only media without antibiotics need be inoculated. See p. 209 for further discussion of specimen processing.

For culturing of blood for fungus, see p. 209.

If an aerobic actinomycete (e.g., *Nocardia* sp.) is suspected, inoculate Middlebrook 7H11 agar; occasional isolates may not grow well on SDA. If actinomycosis is suspected, the specimen must be cultured for anaerobes.

If *Histoplasma capsulatum*, *Blastomyces dermatitidis*, or *Coccidioides immitis* is suspected in a heavily contaminated specimen, yeast extract phosphate medium with ammonia (p. 252) should also be inoculated.

When culturing skin scrapings, hair, or nails, dermatophyte test medium (p. 242) should be inoculated.

The optimal temperature for growth of most clinically encountered fungi is 30°C. If a 30°C incubator is not available, cultures should be incubated at room temperature (approximately 25°C). There is no advantage to simultaneously incubating routine primary cultures at 35–37°C; this should be reserved for when there is reason to suspect the presence of thermally dimorphic organisms or one of the few fungi that prefer the higher temperature. If the incubator is not well humidified, it is advisable to place pans of water near the cultures.

Most cultures should be incubated for 4 weeks before being considered negative for fungus. Cultures for yeasts in oral thrush or vaginitis need to be held only 7 days; cultures suspected of containing thermally dimorphic fungi should be incubated 8 weeks before being reported as negative.

## Macroscopic Examination of Cultures

After initial inoculation and incubation, media should be examined every 2–3 days for growth of fungus. Rapid growers will appear by the first or second time the culture tubes are checked, whereas slow growing fungi may not be evident for 2–3 weeks or longer. It is imperative that any yeast, mold, or actinomycete that grows on a primary medium be subcultured immediately to ensure the viability and isolation of the organism. When mature growth has developed on Sabouraud dextrose agar (SDA), the texture and surface color of the colony should be carefully noted. The color of the reverse (underside) of the colony must also be recorded, along with any pigment that diffuses into the medium. If growth is enhanced on enriched medium, that fact should be noted and a thermally dimorphic fungus should be suspected. It is also helpful to observe whether the fungus grows on medium containing cycloheximide.

To ensure the cultivation of all fungi in a specimen (especially the slower growing pathogens), it is advisable in many cases to hold the cultures for at least a month even though some fungi may have been isolated. When more than one fungus is seen on the slant, a carefully streaked plate is usually necessary for isolation. The lid may be taped closed in several places for safety and prevention of dehydration, but care must be taken not to create anaerobic conditions. Shrink seals are perfect for this situation. As previously mentioned, to prevent dehydration of plates, they should contain 40 ml of agar and a pan of water should be placed in the incubator. If *Coccidioides immitis* is suspected, plates should NOT be used.

## Microscopic Examination of Growth

It is best to examine a fungus microscopically when the culture first begins to grow and form conidia or spores and again a few days later. In many instances the manner of conidiation or sporulation, which is so important to identification, is obscured in old cultures. Potato flake agar often promotes conidiation/sporulation better than does SDA.

There are several methods for microscopically examining a fungus culture. They are:

A. **Tease mount.** Place a drop of lactophenol cotton blue (LPCB) on a clean glass slide. With a bent dissecting needle, remove a small portion of the colony from the agar surface and place it in the drop of LPCB. With two dissecting needles, gently tease apart the mycelial mass of the colony on the slide, cover with a coverslip, and observe under the microscope with low power (100x) and high dry (430x) magnifications. Unfortunately, this method does not always preserve the original position and structure of the conidia, spores, and the like, but it is a very rapid method and always worth a try.

B. **Cellophane tape mount.** Another rapid method of studying the microscopic morphology of a mold is with the aid of clear cellophane tape. Loop back on itself a 1½-in. (~4-cm) strip of clear tape, sticky side out, and hold the tip of the loop securely with a forceps. Press the lower, sticky side very firmly to the surface of the fungal colony and then pull the tape gently away; aerial hyphae will adhere to the tape. Then, with the tape strip opened up, place it on a small drop of LPCB on a glass slide so that the entire sticky side adheres to the slide, and examine it under the microscope. This method is usually successful in retaining the original position of the characteristic fungal structures but has the drawback of requiring the organism be grown on plated medium.

C. **Slide culture.** The best method for preserving and observing the actual structure of a fungus is the slide culture. It is not a rapid technique, but it is unsurpassed as a routine means of studying the fine points of the microscopic morphology of fungi. (Always do a tease mount before a slide culture; organisms suspected of being *Histoplasma*, *Blastomyces*, or *Coccidioides* spp. or *Xylohypha bantiana* should NOT be set up on slide culture.)

The procedure is carried out as follows:

1. Cover the inside bottom of a 100-mm-diameter sterile petri dish with a piece of filter paper.

2. Place a bent glass rod, two pieces of plastic tubing (about 6 cm long, 5 cm apart) or the bending end of a flexible drinking straw in the petri dish.

3. Place a clean, flamed glass microscope slide on the glass rod, plastic tubing, or bent straw.

4. From a plate of SDA (or other agar when desired) poured 4 mm deep, cut a 1 × 1 cm block with a sterile scalpel. Transfer the block to the center of the glass slide.

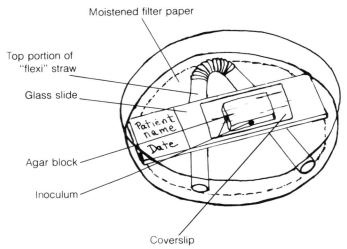

Moistened filter paper

Top portion of "flexi" straw

Glass slide

Patient name
Date

Agar block

Inoculum

Coverslip

5. With a heavy nichrome wire needle (22 gauge) or sterile applicator stick, inoculate the fungus onto the center of the four sides of the agar block.

6. Place a flamed coverslip over the block and apply slight pressure to ensure adherence.

7. Place approximately 1.5 ml of sterile water in the bottom of the petri dish, replace the dish cover, and incubate at room temperature.

8. Examine periodically for growth and add water if the plate begins to dry out. The fungus will ordinarily grow on the surface of the slide and also on the undersurface of the coverslip. The closed petri dish can be placed on the microscope stage and the slide culture can be examined with the low power (10x) objective.

9. When reproductive structures are well developed, use forceps to carefully remove the coverslip and place it on a drop of LPCB on a second slide.

10. With a heavy needle or applicator stick, gently flip the agar block off the original slide into a container of antifungal disinfectant. Place a drop of LPCB on the slide and place a new coverslip over it.

11. Both microscopic preparations from steps 9 and 10 can be sealed around the edges with nail polish or mounting fluid and kept indefinitely for further study or as teaching aids. These slide preparations have been found to last longer if they are stored in a flat position rather than standing on their sides. Huber's modified LPCB with polyvinyl alcohol (p. 231) has been used by the author and is definitely the best method available for preserving slide preparations.

## Procedure for Identification of Yeasts

**A.** Perform germ tube test (p. 219). Only *Candida albicans* and *Candida stellatoidea* will produce germ tubes in serum within 3 h, and they can be differentiated (if desired) by a sucrose assimilation test.

If the result of the germ tube test is negative, continue as follows.

**B.** Be sure that the culture is pure; if doubtful, streak plated medium for isolation. When the culture is pure, inoculate:

    **1.** Assimilation media. Today most laboratories use commercially prepared systems for assimilation and other identification tests; the most commonly used are:

        API 20C (bioMerieux Vitek, Hazelwood, Mo.)

        Minitek (BBL, Cockeysville, Md.)

        Uni-Yeast-Tek (Remel, Lenexa, Kans.)

        Vitek Yeast Biochemical Card (bioMerieux Vitek, Hazelwood, Mo.)

        Yeast Identification Panel (MicroScan, Sacramento, Calif.)

    **2.** Cornmeal-Tween 80 agar plate (p. 241); this or another yeast morphology agar should accompany all biochemical identification systems.

**C.** If an acceptable identification is not obtained, subsequent tests may be required for:

    fermentation (p. 243)

    appearance of isolate in Sabouraud broth (p. 248)

    inhibition of isolate by cycloheximide

    urease activity, if not included in the commercial system (p. 251)

    phenoloxidase (caffeic acid disk, p. 219)

**D.** Consult Tables 4.1–4.4 (pp. 64, 66, 76, and 79) for identification of genus and species.

## Isolation of Yeast When Mixed with Bacteria

Yeasts often grow mixed with bacteria on primary culture. It is absolutely essential that only pure cultures be used in assimilation, fermentation, and other biochemical tests for identification.

Careful streaking of the organisms onto plated medium with or without antibiotics often yields isolated colonies. If the yeast is sensitive to cycloheximide, inhibitory mold agar (p. 245) should be used. Persistent bacterial contamination may be eliminated with the following acidification method.

Place 10 ml of Sabouraud dextrose broth in each of four tubes

To tube no. 1, add 1 drop of 1 N HCl

To tube no. 2, add 2 drops of 1 N HCl

To tube no. 3, add 3 drops of 1 N HCl

To tube no. 4, add 4 drops of 1 N HCl

Make a suspension of the yeast-bacteria mixture in sterile water. Add a drop of the suspension to each of the four Sabouraud dextrose broth-HCl tubes. Incubate at 25–30°C for 24 h.

Subculture a loopful of broth from each tube to plated media and incubate for 48 h.

In most instances, there will have been an acid concentration at which the bacteria were inhibited and the yeast was allowed to grow.

## Germ Tube Test for the Presumptive Identification of *Candida albicans*

1.  Make a very light suspension of a yeastlike organism in 0.5–1.0 ml of sterile serum. The optimum inoculum is $10^5$–$10^6$ cells per ml; an increased concentration of inoculum causes a significant decrease in the percentage of cells forming germ tubes. Pooled human serum can be used as well as animal sera or a variety of media. A clean Pasteur pipette tip can be used to inoculate the serum and can be left in the tube during incubation.
2.  Incubate at 35–37°C for no longer than 3 h.
3.  Place one drop of the yeast-serum mixture on a slide with a coverslip. Examine microscopically for germ tube production.

A known strain of *Candida albicans* should be tested with each new batch of serum.

Germ tubes are the beginnings of true hyphae and appear as filaments that are NOT constricted at their point of origin on the parent cell.

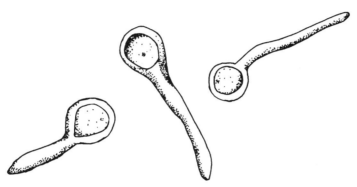

## Rapid Enzyme Tests for the Presumptive Identification of *Candida albicans*

Several systems (Murex *C. albicans* [Murex Diagnostics, Norcross, Ga.], Bacti-Card Candida [Remel, Lenexa, Kans.], and Albicans-Sure [Clinical Standards Laboratories, Rancho Dominguez, Calif.]) are now commercially available for the rapid (5 to 30 min) presumptive identification of *Candida albicans* in culture. Each system utilizes two substrates for the detection of beta-galactosamidase and L-proline aminopeptidase. Of the clinically encountered yeasts, only *C. albicans* produces both of these enzymes. Evaluations of the systems show them to be rapid, acceptable alternatives to the germ tube test. Manufacturers' instructions must be followed.

## Caffeic Acid Disk Test

Caffeic acid is one of several good substrates for the detection of phenoloxidase enzyme activity. When phenoloxidase is present, the caffeic acid is broken down to melanin, resulting in a dark brown to black color. As *Cryptococcus neoformans* is the only clinically encountered yeast that produces phenoloxidase, the test is extremely useful for identification and/or confirmation of this organism. Although birdseed agar may also be used, the advantages of this disk test are speed and improved reliability. See procedure on following page.

1. Culture the isolated yeast on cornmeal-Tween 80 agar. Because phenoloxidase is inhibited by glucose, it is essential that the growth medium be glucose free; cornmeal-Tween 80 agar is usually the most readily available medium to meet this requirement.
2. Place a caffeic acid disk (available from Remel, Lenexa, Kans.) on a glass slide. Moisten the disk with 30–40 µl of water.
3. Inoculate the disk with several colonies of the isolated yeast.
4. Incubate the disk at 22 to 35°C in a moist chamber.
5. Read for development of brown to black pigment. Most positive reactions are seen within 30 min, but the test should be held at least 4 h before being considered negative. On rare occasions, an organism may require several generations of growth on cornmeal agar before the enzyme can be detected.

## Conversion of Thermally Dimorphic Fungi in Culture

A mycelial colony that is morphologically suggestive of a thermally dimorphic fungus at room temperature must also be grown in its yeastlike form at 35–37°C to confirm its identification. This is essential, as there are several monomorphic molds that resemble the filamentous phase of thermally dimorphic fungi. In addition, the mold forms of some dimorphic fungi may not be definitive microscopically, and the yeast phase can serve to identify them.

These organisms MUST be handled in a biological safety cabinet. To test for the ability of a mycelial form to convert to a yeast phase:

1. Inoculate mycelial growth onto a fresh moist slant of brain heart infusion agar in a screw-cap tube. A small amount of brain heart infusion broth added to the tube ensures sufficient moisture. After the fragment of mold inoculum has been emulsified in the moisture, pull it up and place it on the agar slant.
2. Incubate at 35–37°C. Keep the screw cap closed tightly to retain the moisture, but loosen it daily to allow the colony to "breathe."
3. Periodically examine the slant and make a wet preparation of any yeastlike area.
4. If only a mycelial form grows, transfer it to another moistened brain heart infusion slant and incubate again at 35–37°C. It may be necessary to make several serial transfers to attain complete conversion to the yeast phase.

In some instances, in vitro conversion is exceedingly difficult or slow, and exoantigen tests or DNA probes may be preferred or required to confirm identification. Manufacturer's instructions (GenProbe, San Diego, Calif.) should be followed for performing DNA probe tests. For complete instructions on performing the exoantigen test, see Isenberg, 1992, pp. 6.11.10–6.11.12.

## Method of Inducing Sporulation of *Apophysomyces elegans* and *Saksenaea vasiformis* (Padhye and Ajello, 1988)

This procedure is recommended for use in identifying all nonsporulating zygomycetes isolated from clinical specimens. The growth on SDA at 25°C should consist of broad, nonseptate to sparsely septate, branched, hyaline hyphae without sporangial formation.

1. Grow the isolate on an SDA plate at 25°C for 1 week.
2. Aseptically cut out a 1-cm agar block permeated with the hyphal growth.
3. Transfer the block to a petri plate containing 20 ml of sterile distilled water and 0.2 ml of filter-sterilized 10% yeast extract. Shrink-seal plates to prevent spillage.
4. Incubate the blocks in the water solution at 35–37°C (lower temperature will yield fewer or no sporangia). After 5 days of incubation, a thin film of growth should appear over the surface of the water.
5. Make wet preparations (with lactophenol cotton blue) of portions of the film on days 5, 10, and 15 of incubation. Examine microscopically for sporangia. See p. 112 and 114 for descriptions of *A. elegans* and *S. vasiformis*, respectively.

## In Vitro Hair Perforation Test (for differentiation of *Trichophyton mentagrophytes* and *Trichophyton rubrum*)

1. Place 1-cm-long fragments of healthy human hair in a petri plate or tube. Sterilize by autoclaving at 15 lb/in² for 15 min. The clearest and fastest results are obtained with light colored hair from a child (less than 12 years old). Adult hair will give correct results if the hair has not been exposed to hair spray or a combination of bleach and permanent wave (Salkin et al., 1985b).
2. In a sterile 50-ml screw-cap tube, place 8–10 of the sterile hair fragments; add 20–25 ml of sterile distilled water and 0.1 ml of 10% filter-sterilized yeast extract. (Plastic conical tubes used for concentrating specimens for acid-fast bacilli work well; tubes have proven safer to handle than petri plates when doing this test.)
3. Place several fragments of the fungal culture into the tube.
4. Incubate at room temperature for 4 weeks or until a positive reaction is seen (average, 8–10 days). Examine at weekly intervals by placing one or two hairs from the culture onto a slide with a drop of lactophenol cotton blue and coverslip. Look for wedge-shaped perforations caused by hyphae that penetrate the hairs perpendicularly.

The hair is perforated by *T. mentagrophytes* but not by *T. rubrum* (see Table 6.7, p. 172).

Positive in vitro hair perforation test

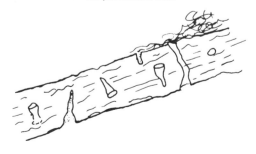

## Germ Tube Test for Differentiation of Some Dematiaceous Fungi

Germ tube formation plays an important role in identification of the genera of dematiaceous fungi that form macroconidia with transverse septa, i.e., *Bipolaris*, *Drechslera*, and *Exserohilum* spp.

1. Place a drop of water on a microscope slide.
2. Inoculate the drop of water with a small amount of the actively growing fungus. Examine the slide microscopically to confirm that conidia are present.
3. Place a coverslip over the suspension.
4. Incubate in a moist chamber at room temperature for 8 to 24 h.
5. Examine the slide microscopically to determine the origin and orientation of the germ tubes. See Table 6.6 (p. 150) for interpretation of results.

## Maintenance of Stock Fungal Cultures

### OIL OVERLAY TECHNIQUE

Obtain a small but actively growing fungal culture on a short slant of SDA. Pour over it a good grade of sterile heavy mineral oil (Saybolt viscosity 330 at 100°F, autoclaved at 15 lb/in² for 45 min in half-filled 250-ml flasks). It is absolutely necessary that the oil cover not only the fungal colony but also the whole agar surface; otherwise the exposed agar will act as a wick and in time cause the medium to dry out and the colony to die.

The stock cultures are stored upright at room temperature, and most will remain viable for several years. Unfortunately, some fungi must be transferred very often, as they are difficult to keep alive.

To transfer a fungus from an oiled culture, remove a small portion of the colony with a long, disposable inoculating needle or a sterile applicator stick. Drain off the oil along the inside of the tube and place the inoculum on a fresh agar slant.

### WATER CULTURE TECHNIQUE

Rub a sterile moistened swab over the surface of an actively conidiating/sporulating fungus colony; wash the swab off into a screw-cap tube containing approximately 4 ml of sterile distilled water. Tighten the cap and store at room temperature. Add sterile distilled water periodically if any evaporation occurs.

To prepare a subculture, shake the water culture to resuspend the fungus. Open the tube, flame the mouth, and with a sterile Pasteur pipette transfer approximately 0.4 ml of the suspension to a slant of SDA. Incubate the SDA at 25–30°C.

### FREEZING TECHNIQUE

Culture the fungus on a slant of potato dextrose agar in a screw-cap glass test tube. Incubate at 25–30°C until the organism reaches maturity and is actively producing conidia or spores. Close caps tightly and place tubes into a freezer. Best results are obtained at −70°C, but −20°C has also been used with success. If stored at −20°C, organisms may need to be subcultured annually.

To subculture, remove the tube from the freezer and chip a small portion of the colony from the agar slant. Place the chipped section on a fresh agar slant and immediately return the frozen slant to the freezer. If the culture is allowed to thaw, it should not be refrozen; the fungus must be transferred to a fresh slant, incubated to maturity, and then frozen.

# Staining Methods

# 8

Positive and negative controls must be run on new lots of stain and periodically thereafter. If the stain is not frequently used, it is advisable to run controls each time the staining procedure is performed on an unknown organism.

## Acid-Fast Stains

### MODIFIED KINYOUN METHOD FOR *NOCARDIA* SPP.

The filaments of *Nocardia* spp. usually appear at least partially acid fast with this staining procedure. Acid-fast organisms stain pink to red.

**A.** Procedure

    **1.** Make a smear and fix over flame.

    **2.** Flood slide with Kinyoun carbol-fuchsin for 5 min.

    **3.** Pour off excess stain.

    **4.** Flood slide with 50% alcohol and immediately wash with water.

    **5.** Decolorize with 1% aqueous sulfuric acid (see alternate decolorizer below).

6. Wash with tap water.
7. Counterstain with methylene blue or brilliant green for 1 min.
8. Rinse with water, dry, and examine under oil-immersion objective.

Negative and positive controls should be included each time this method is used.

B. Reagents
1. Kinyoun carbol-fuchsin (same as for staining mycobacteria)

> Basic fuchsin ................................. 4 g
> Phenol ......................................... 8 ml
> Alcohol, 95% ............................... 20 ml
> Distilled water ............................ 100 ml

Dissolve the dye in the alcohol and then add the water and phenol.

2. 1% aqueous $H_2SO_4$ (see alternative decolorizer below)

> Concentrated $H_2SO_4$ ...................... 1 ml
> Distilled water .............................. 99 ml

Be sure to add the acid to the water, not vice versa.

3. Counterstain

> Methylene blue .......................... 2.5 g
> Ethanol, 95% ........................... 100.0 ml
> or
> Brilliant green ........................... 0.5 g
> Distilled water ......................... 100.0 ml

Use of the following decolorizing agent, commonly used in the fluorochrome method for acid-fast bacilli, may be successfully used to substitute for steps 4 and 5 of the above procedure:

> Concentrated HCl ...................... 0.5 ml
> Ethanol, 70% ........................... 99.5 ml

## ACID-FAST STAIN FOR ASCOSPORES
When staining for ascospores, the classic Kinyoun method is used (as for mycobacteria), i.e., decolorize with solution of:

> Concentrated HCL ...................... 3 ml
> Ethanol, 95% .............................. 97 ml

Add acid to water, mix well.
The ascospores will stain red; other cells will take the counterstain.

## ASCOSPORE STAIN

1. Culture the fungus on a medium that promotes ascospore formation (see p. 234).
2. Make thin smear and fix in flame.
3. Stain with 5% aqueous malachite green (filter before using), containing Tergitol 7 (Sigma Chemical Co., St. Louis, Mo.) for 3 min.
4. Wash with tap water.
5. Decolorize with 95% ethyl alcohol for 30 s.
6. Wash with tap water.
7. Counterstain with 5% aqueous safranin for 30 s.
8. Wash with water, allow to dry, and examine under oil immersion objective.

Ascospores stain green and vegetative cells stain red.

The acid-fast stain (p. 226) is also useful for observing ascospores. It should be noted that ascospores may be observed in simple aqueous wet mounts without any stain.

## CALCOFLUOR WHITE STAIN

A relatively new stain that has been found to be extremely useful in the clinical mycology laboratory is Calcofluor white. Calcofluor white binds to beta 1–3 and 1–4 polysaccharides such as cellulose and chitin (present in fungal cell walls) and fluoresces when exposed to UV radiation. It is exceedingly useful for direct microscopic examination of specimens, as the fungal elements are seen much more easily than with the older traditional potassium hydroxide (KOH) preparations.

### Preparation of stain solution

| | |
|---|---|
| Calcofluor white M2R* .............. | 100 mg |
| Evans Blue ............................ | 50 mg |
| Distilled water .......................... | 100 ml |

*Commercially available from Sigma Chemical Co. and Polysciences, Inc.

Mix well. Store at room temperature in a dark bottle.

### Procedure

Smear specimen on glass slide; specimen may be stained while wet but must be allowed to dry and quickly heat fixed if the slide is to be subsequently reprocessed with another stain.

Add one drop of Calcofluor white stain solution. One drop of 10% KOH may also be added if clearing is required.

Apply coverslip. Allow slide to sit at room temperature approximately 3 min. (Periodically prepare and examine smears of known fungi to ensure quality of the reagent, procedure, and microscope.)

Examine slide with a UV microscope that is equipped with an excitation filter that transmits wavelengths between 300 and 412 nm (maximum absorbance of Calcofluor white is 347 nm) and a barrier filter that removes UV while transmitting visible blue light and longer wavelengths. The required light source is a mercury vapor lamp; quartz halogen bulbs are usually not suitable, as the energy output is too low.

Fungal elements will stand out as bright apple green on a red background or white on a blue background, depending on the barrier filter used.

If the slide is to be saved or restained, remove the coverslip, rinse the slide briefly with distilled water, and air dry. The slide can later be restained with Calcofluor white or other stains such as Gomori methenamine silver, Gram, etc.

## GIEMSA STAIN

The Giemsa stain is used for the detection of intracellular *Histoplasma capsulatum* in bone marrow or blood smears. The blood smears are made from the buffy coat of centrifuged citrated blood or from the bottom of the tube, where heavily infected cells are often found. *H. capsulatum* is seen as small, oval yeast cells that stain light to dark blue with a hyaline halo due to the unstained cell wall (see p. 14). Giemsa stain is commercially available.

1. Place slide in 100% methanol for 1 min (to fix smear).
2. Drain off methanol.
3. Flood slide with Giemsa stain (freshly diluted 1:10 with distilled water) for 5 min.
4. Wash with water; air dry.

## GOMORI METHENAMINE SILVER STAIN

Of the special stains for fungi, methenamine silver nitrate is considered by many to be the most useful for screening clinical specimens. It provides better contrast and often stains fungal elements that may not be revealed by other procedures. Fungi are sharply delineated in black against a pale green background. The inner parts of hyphae are charcoal gray. Certain bacteria (including *Nocardia* spp.) as well as some tissue elements also take the stain, so it must be remembered that all that is gray or black is not necessarily a fungus.

Histology laboratories routinely perform some method of Gomori methenamine silver staining. The following simpler and faster method (Mahan and Sale, 1978) may also be used on smeared material or deparaffinized tissue.

**Solutions required (all are aqueous solutions)**
 10% chromic acid (chromium trioxide)
  5% silver nitrate
  3% methenamine (hexamethylenetetramine)
  5% borax (sodium borate)
  1% gold chloride
  1% sodium metabisulfite
  5% sodium thiosulfate

## Preparation of stains
Methenamine silver nitrate solution

      3% methenamine ........................... 40 ml
      5% silver nitrate ........................... 2 ml
      5% borax ..................................... 3 ml
      Distilled water ............................. 35 ml

This solution must be freshly prepared when ready to use; it can be used only once. The other solutions may be reused for up to one month provided fungal contamination does not occur.

## Light green
STOCK SOLUTION

      Light green SF-yellowish .............. 0.2 g
      Distilled water ......................... 100.0 ml
      Glacial acetic acid ....................... 0.2 ml

Solution is stable for one year.

WORKING SOLUTION

      Stock light green solution ............. 10 ml
      Distilled water ............................. 40 ml

Solution is stable for one month.

## Procedure
Before starting, heat Coplin jar of methenamine silver nitrate solution in oven or water bath until the solution becomes a deep golden brown (approximately 95°C). Then,

**A.** If slide to be stained is paraffin fixed, rehydrate (see procedure, p. 232); other slides must be fixed by heating or submerging in alcohol. Positive control slides must be included each time the staining procedure is performed.

**B.** Rinse slides with water.

**C.** Place slides in reagents in Coplin jars as follows:

    **1.** Chromic acid (discard after use) ........................... 10 min
    **2.** Running tap water ................................... 5 s
    **3.** 1% sodium metabisulfite ......................... 1 min
    **4.** Hot tap water ........................................ 1 min
    **5.** Methenamine silver nitrate solution,
        approximately 95°C. ......................... 5–10 min

Periodically remove control slide, wash with water, and observe microscopically to determine when optimal staining has been achieved. The color should never be so intense as to obscure the morphologic detail of a fungus. Prolonged staining time may be required when old and nonviable fungal elements or filaments of actinomycetes are suspected.

  **6.** When control shows optimal staining, rinse all slides in hot tap water and then in gradually cooler water.
  **7.** Distilled water .................................................... Rinse
  **8.** 1% gold chloride ................................................. 10 s
  **9.** Distilled water .................................................... Rinse
  **10.** 5% sodium thiosulfate ......................................... 3 min
  **11.** Running tap water ............................................... 30 s
  **12.** Light green working solution ............................... 30 s

**D.** Rinse twice with each increasing concentration of ethanol: 70%, 95%, and absolute alcohol.
**E.** Dip slides twice in xylene.
**F.** Place drop of mounting medium on slide and cover with coverslip.

## GRAM STAIN (Hucker Modification)
Fungi are gram positive but often stain poorly.

**A.** Procedure
  **1.** Fix the smear by passing it over a flame.
  **2.** Place crystal violet solution on the slide for 20 s.
  **3.** Wash gently with tap water.
  **4.** Apply Gram iodine solution to the slide for 20 s.
  **5.** Wash gently with tap water.
  **6.** Decolorize quickly in solution of equal parts of acetone and 95% ethanol.
  **7.** Wash gently with tap water.
  **8.** Counterstain with safranin for 10 s.
  **9.** Wash with tap water; air dry or blot dry.
**B.** Reagents
  **1.** Crystal violet solution
    **a.** Crystal violet, 85% dye content ........................................ 2 g
    Ethyl alcohol, 95% ...................................................... 10 ml
    Dissolve the dye in alcohol.
    Add distilled water .................................................... 100 ml
    **b.** Ammonium oxalate ..................................................... 4 g
    Distilled water ........................................................... 400 ml
    Dissolve the ammonium oxalate in the water.
   Mix the crystal violet-alcohol solution (a) with the ammonium oxalate solution (b).
  **2.** Gram iodine solution
   Iodine ........................................................................... 1 g
   Potassium iodide ............................................................ 2 g
   Dissolve the iodine and potassium iodide completely in 5 ml of distilled water.
   Add distilled water ........................................................ 240 ml

Sodium bicarbonate, 5% aqueous solution ....................... 60 ml
    (i.e., 3 g of NaHCO$_3$ + 57 ml of distilled water)
Mix well; store in amber glass bottle.

**3.** Counterstain
Safranin O ...................................................................................... 1 g
Ethyl alcohol, 95% ............................................................... 40 ml
Dissolve the dye in the alcohol.
Add distilled water ............................................................ 400 ml
Mix well.

*Note*: A slide that has been Gram stained can be decolorized by flooding with acetone for 30–60 s and rinsing well with water. Special fungus stains can then be performed on the slide.

## LACTOPHENOL COTTON BLUE

Lactophenol cotton blue is used as both a mounting fluid and a stain. Lactic acid acts as a clearing agent and aids in preserving the fungal structures, phenol acts as a killing agent, glycerol prevents drying, and cotton blue gives a color to the structures.

    Lactic acid ................................... 20 ml
    Phenol crystals ........................... 20 g
      (or phenol, concentrated .......... 20 ml)
    Glycerol (or glycerine) .................. 40 ml
    Distilled water ............................ 20 ml
    Cotton blue .............................. 0.05 g
      (or 1% aqueous solution ............. 2 ml)

Dissolve phenol in the lactic acid, glycerol, and water by gently heating (if crystals are used). Then add cotton blue (Poirrier's blue and aniline blue are analogous to cotton blue).
Mix well.
For use, see p. 216.

## LACTOPHENOL COTTON BLUE WITH POLYVINYL ALCOHOL (PVA)
Huber's PVA mounting medium, modified*

This modification of Huber's plastic mount (Huber and Caplin, 1947) is excellent for making permanent mounts of fungal wet preparations or slide cultures. Upon drying for at least 24 h on a flat surface, these mounts are permanent and will not be dissolved in ether, xylene, or alcohols, and the fixed fungal structures remain picture-perfect for years. See method on next page.

---

*Appreciation is extended to Lawrence M. Bobon of Riverside Hospital in Wilmington, Del., for the updating and reinstatement of Huber's method.

### Reagents

PVA; molecular weight, 70,000–100,000 (Sigma Chemical Co., catalog no. P-1763)

Phenol purified grade (Sigma no. P-5566 or Fisher no. A91 1–500)

Lactic acid, ACS reagent (Sigma no. L-1893)

Aniline blue, certified (Aldrich Chemical Co., catalog no. 86,102–2). This is analogous to cotton blue.

### Preparation

1. Add 7.5 g of PVA powder to 50 ml of cold deionized water in a beaker.
2. Transfer beaker to a heated stirring plate; add a magnetic rod for mixing.
3. Place a thermometer into the beaker to monitor temperature.
4. Add 22 g of lactic acid (BEFORE adding phenol).
5. Add 22 g of phenol crystals (or 22 ml of melted phenol).
6. Add 0.05 g of aniline blue.
7. Heat and stir the solution until the temperature reaches 90°C. Do not boil or go over 100°C.
   Remove from hot plate.
8. Dispense into small dropper bottles (used washed ones from blood bank panel cells work well). Tighten dropper bottle caps and store at room temperature.

### Procedure

Place one drop of PVA mounting fluid on a slide with a sample of fungal growth. Apply coverslip. Allow to dry on a flat surface. Huber's modified PVA mounting medium may be used as a replacement for lactophenol cotton blue. Care must be taken to avoid coverslip runover or droppings on the bench top since they are difficult to remove. While the solution is in liquid form it can be cleaned from surfaces with water; after drying, a razor blade is required to remove the hardened material.

Slides can be examined microscopically at low or high dry power as soon as the slides are prepared. After adequate drying time (2 to 4 days), the slides can be examined under oil immersion, cleansed in xylene, or decontaminated by dipping in disinfectant.

## REHYDRATION OF PARAFFIN-EMBEDDED TISSUE

Treat slides as follows.

Xylene (in Coplin jar) .................. 12 min
Repeat, using two more jars of xylene
Absolute ethanol ................. Rinse twice
95% ethanol ........................ Rinse twice
70% ethanol ........................ Rinse twice
Distilled water ..................... Rinse twice

Proceed with staining procedure.

# Media

Many of the media prepared for mycology are used relatively rarely in the typical clinical microbiology laboratory. Freshness during long storage may be maintained by dispensing agar media into screw-cap tubes, autoclaving, allowing it to cool as butts, and storing it in the refrigerator. When needed, the appropriate number of butts are melted in a boiling water bath and then poured into petri plates or allowed to cool as slants.

Whenever a new batch of medium is placed in use, positive and negative control organisms must be tested. If the medium is not often used, it is advisable to run controls each time an unknown organism is tested.

# Ascospore Media
## ACETATE ASCOSPORE AGAR

| | |
|---|---|
| Potassium acetate | 5.00 g |
| Yeast extract | 1.25 g |
| Dextrose | 0.50 g |
| Agar | 15.00 g |
| Distilled water | 500.00 ml |

Dissolve by boiling for 1 min; dispense in screw-cap tubes.
Autoclave (15 lb/in²) for 15 min.
Allow tubes to cool in slanted position or as butts to be melted and slanted as needed.

## GORODKOWA MEDIUM

| | |
|---|---|
| Dextrose | 1.25 g |
| NaCl | 2.60 g |
| Beef extract | 5.00 g |
| Agar | 5.00 g |
| Distilled water | 500.00 ml |

Dispense into screw-cap tubes.
Autoclave (15 lb/in²) for 15 min.
Allow to harden as slants or as butts to be melted and slanted as needed.

## V-8 MEDIUM FOR ASCOSPORES

| | |
|---|---|
| V-8 vegetable juice | 500 ml |
| Dry yeast | 10 g |
| Agar | 20 g |
| Distilled water | 500 ml |

Dissolve agar in water by boiling.
Mix vegetable juice and dry yeast, adjust to pH 6.8 with 20% KOH, add to agar-water mixture, and mix well.
Dispense into screw-cap tube.
Autoclave (15 lb/in²) for 15 min.
Allow to cool as slants or as butts to be melted and slanted as needed.

## Assimilation Media (for Yeasts)*

Assimilation is the utilization of a carbon (or nitrogen) source by a microorganism in the presence of oxygen. A positive reaction is indicated by the presence of growth or a pH shift in the medium.

## I. WICKERHAM BROTH METHOD

### Carbon assimilation medium

> Yeast nitrogen base .................... 6.70 g
> Appropriate carbohydrate ........... 5.00 g
> Distilled water ........................ 100.00 ml

If necessary, heat to dissolve.

Sterilize by Seitz or membrane filter.

Add 0.5 ml of the solution to 4.5 ml of sterile distilled water in screw-cap tubes.

These tubes may now be stored in the refrigerator, ready for use, for one month.

*Note*: Care must be taken to ensure that carbon compounds are pure and not mixed with other carbohydrates. It is advisable to check each new lot of a carbon compound with control yeasts that can and cannot assimilate it before using the material in assimilation studies. The sugars most commonly employed are listed in Tables 4.2–4.4 (pp. 66, 76, and 79).

### Nitrate assimilation medium

> Yeast carbon base .................... 11.70 g
> Potassium nitrate (KNO$_3$) ............ 0.78 g
> Distilled water ........................ 100.00 ml

Warm gently to dissolve.

Sterilize by Seitz or membrane filtration.

Add 0.5 ml of medium to 4.5 ml of sterile distilled water in screw-cap tubes.

These tubes may be stored in the refrigerator for one month.

Tubes of yeast nitrogen base without sugar and yeast carbon base without KNO$_3$ should be prepared and used as controls to check "carryover" of nutrients that may have been stored within the yeast cell when grown on the previous medium.

### Procedure

1. Make a suspension of the yeast in sterile distilled water. This suspension should not exceed the turbidity of McFarland no. 1 standard (prepared by mixing 0.1 ml of 1% barium chloride with 9.9 ml of 1% sulfuric acid).

---

*Most clinical laboratories now use commercially prepared systems for assimilation tests; see p. 218 for a list of those available.

2. Add 0.1–0.2 ml of the yeast suspension to each tube of medium. Include a tube of yeast nitrogen base without any carbon source and a tube of yeast carbon base without KNO$_3$ as controls for carryover.

3. Incubate tubes at the yeast's optimal temperature. If the organism grows at 35–37°C, positive reactions are usually more rapid at this temperature. Shaking the culture tubes will also enhance growth.

4. Examine cultures over a period of 7–14 days for dense turbidity caused by growth.

5. The negative control tubes without carbon or nitrogen source should show no growth. If growth is present, the test is invalid because of carryover. In such cases, a small amount of growth from each tube should be transferred to another tube of the same medium and the test should be repeated.

For identification of yeasts, see Tables 4.2–4.4 (pp. 66, 76, and 79).

## II. AUXANOGRAPHIC PLATE METHOD (HALEY AND STANDARD MODIFICATION)

**For carbon assimilation tests**

> Yeast nitrogen base .................... 0.67 g
> Noble or washed agar .............. 20.00 g
> Distilled water .................... 1,000.00 ml

Dispense in 20-ml quantities into 18 × 150 mm screw-cap tubes.
Autoclave (15 lb/in²) for 15 min.
Allow to harden as butts. Store in refrigerator.

PROCEDURE

1. Melt a tube of nitrogen base medium in a boiling water bath; allow to cool to 47–48°C.

2. With a sterile cotton-tipped applicator, make a heavy suspension of a 24- to 72-h yeast culture in 4 ml of sterile distilled water. The density should equal that of a McFarland no. 4 or no. 5 standard.

3. Pour the yeast suspension into the tube of molten yeast nitrogen base agar. Mix very thoroughly by inverting tube several times.

4. Pour the yeast-agar mixture into a sterile 15 × 150 mm petri dish. Allow to solidify at room temperature.

5. Place carbohydrate disks (available from BBL Microbiology Systems, Cockeysville, Md., and Difco Laboratories, Detroit, Mich.), evenly spaced, on the plate.

6. Incubate at 30°C for 18–24 h and then examine for growth around each disk. Any amount of growth around a disk indicates that the yeast assimilates that sugar. The plates may be reincubated for an additional 24 h, but reincubation is usually not necessary.

**For nitrate assimilation tests**

**A.** Medium

> Yeast carbon base .......................... 12 g
> Noble or washed agar .................... 20 g
> Distilled water .......................... 1,000 ml

Tube in 20-ml aliquots and autoclave at 15 lb/in² for 15 min. Store in refrigerator.

**B.** Peptone solution for positive control

> Peptone ......................................... 10 g
> Distilled water ............................. 100 ml

Sterilize by filtration; store in refrigerator.

PROCEDURE

**1.** Melt a tube of yeast carbon base medium in a boiling water bath; allow to cool to 47–48°C.

**2.** Make an aqueous suspension of the yeast to a density equal to a McFarland no. 1 standard.

**3.** Add 0.1 ml of the yeast suspension to the tube of medium. Mix thoroughly.

**4.** Pour the yeast-agar mixture into a sterile 15 × 100 mm petri dish. Allow to solidify at room temperature.

**5.** Place approximately 1 mg of $KNO_3$ crystals on agar surface away from the center of the plate.

**6.** Place approximately 0.1 ml of peptone solution (positive control) on agar surface opposite the $KNO_3$ site.

**7.** Incubate at 30°C for 48–96 h. Growth must occur in the "peptone area" for test to be valid. If growth is seen in the peptone area, examine for growth in the $KNO_3$ area (growth indicates assimilation of $KNO_3$).

## III. AGAR WITH INDICATOR METHOD

This modification of the Wickerham medium was devised by Adams and Cooper (1974). It is easier to read than the conventional methods, yet it is equally reliable. The medium is in the form of agar slants with an indicator added. It is less troublesome than other formulations, for it can be sterilized by autoclaving after the carbohydrates have been added. The quality of each batch of medium should be tested with standard reference strains of yeasts.

**Basal medium**

> Bromcresol purple (1.6%) ............. 0.2 ml
> 0.1 N NaOH ................................. 1.0 ml
> Noble agar .................................... 2.0 g
> Deionized water ......................... 90.0 ml

Heat to dissolve.

### Stock carbohydrate solution

$$
\begin{array}{lr}
\text{Carbohydrate} & 1.00 \text{ g} \\
\text{(if using raffinose)} & 2.00 \text{ g} \\
\text{Yeast nitrogen base} & 0.67 \text{ g} \\
\text{Deionized water} & 10.00 \text{ ml}
\end{array}
$$

Mix to dissolve; gently heat if necessary.

### Preparation
1. Add the stock carbohydrate solution to the melted agar base.
2. Mix well.
3. Adjust to pH 7.0.
4. Dispense in 5-ml amounts in $16 \times 125$ mm screw-cap tubes.
5. Sterilize by autoclaving at exactly 10 lb/in² for 10 min.
6. Allow to solidify in a slanted position.
7. Store in refrigerator at 4°C.

### Inoculation and incubation
1. Suspend a 2-mm loopful of pure culture in 9 ml of sterile water.
2. Inoculate each assimilation slant with 0.1 ml of the suspension.
3. Incubate at room temperature (25°C), examining at 7 and 14 days for abundant growth and acid production (yellow).

Assimilations are considered negative when there is no significant difference between the growth of the organism on the carbohydrate medium and that on the control medium without carbohydrate.

## Birdseed Agar (Niger Seed Agar)

> Guizotia abyssinica seed ............. 50 mg
> (Commonly known as niger seed; it is
> available at most stores that sell bird
> feed.)
> Distilled water ............................ 100 ml

Pulverize in blender.
Add 900 ml of distilled water.
Boil for 30 min.
Filter through four layers of gauze and then add enough distilled water to make volume 1,000 ml.
Add:

> KH$_2$PO$_4$ ............................................ 1 g
> Creatinine ....................................... 1 g
> Agar ................................................. 15 g
> Chloramphenicol ............................. 1 g

Mix well. Autoclave (15 lb/in$^2$) for 15 min.
Pour into tubes and cool in slanted position or as butts to be melted and slanted as needed.

Inoculate with suspected *Cryptococcus* sp. (fresh isolate) and incubate at room temperature for no more than 7 days.
Only *Cryptococcus neoformans* produces phenoloxidase, which breaks down the substrate, resulting in the production of melanin and the development of dark brown to black colonies. Colonies of other yeasts are cream to beige.
Chemically defined tests such as the caffeic acid disk test also detect phenoloxidase and have the advantage of rapidness and sensitivity; see p. 219.

## Brain Heart Infusion Agar

This medium is recommended for the cultivation of fastidious pathogenic fungi such as *Histoplasma capsulatum* and *Blastomyces dermatitidis*.

> Brain heart infusion agar
> (dehydrated) ............................. 52 g
> Distilled water ......................... 1,000 ml

Dissolve ingredients by boiling.
Dispense into screw-cap tubes; autoclave (15 lb/in$^2$) for 15 min.
Cool in slanted position with 1-in. (2.5-cm) butt.
Store in refrigerator.
The antibiotics cycloheximide and chloramphenicol may be added to this medium in the same manner that they are added to Sabouraud dextrose agar. This selective form of the medium is sometimes helpful in isolating fastidious pathogenic fungi when bacteria and saprophytic fungi are also present. In such cases, yeast extract-phosphate agar with ammonia (p. 252) is recommended.

## Casein Agar
(For differentiation of aerobic actinomycetes and characterization of some dematiaceous fungi)

### SOLUTION A

> Skim milk (dehydrated or instant
>     nonfat dry milk) ......................... 10 g
> Distilled water ............................... 90 ml

Add milk with constant stirring to avoid lumping.

### SOLUTION B

> Agar ............................................. 3 g
> Distilled water ............................... 97 ml

Autoclave each solution separately at 15 lb/in$^2$ for 10 min.

Cool both solutions to 45–50°C and then combine solutions and mix well.

Pour into petri plates (or into screw-cap tubes and allow to solidify as butts to be melted and poured as needed).

Inoculate a 10-mm area heavily with a pure culture. Include positive and negative control cultures. Three or four organisms can be tested on one 100-mm plate if they are evenly spaced. Incubate at room temperature or 37°C for 2 weeks. Examine every few days for clearing (hydrolysis) of casein around or directly beneath the colony.

For results with aerobic actinomycetes, see Table 3.1 (p. 56).

For results with dematiaceous fungi, see Table 6.5 (p. 138).

## Cornmeal Agar

Cornmeal ..................................... 40 g
Agar ............................................ 20 g
Tween 80 (polysorbate 80) ............ 10 ml
Distilled water ......................... 1,000 ml

Mix cornmeal well with 500 ml of water; heat to 65°C for 1 h.
Filter through gauze and then paper until clear. Restore to original volume.
Adjust to pH 6.6–6.8. Add agar dissolved in 500 ml of water.
Add Tween 80. Autoclave (15 lb/in²) for 15 min.
Dispense into petri dishes or into screw-cap tubes to form butts to be melted and poured as needed.

Cornmeal with Tween 80 is used in distinguishing the different genera of yeasts and the various species of *Candida* and can also be useful in slide cultures, as it stimulates conidiation in many fungi. If 10 g of dextrose is added to the medium in place of the Tween 80, the medium can be used to differentiate *Trichophyton mentagrophytes* from *Trichophyton rubrum* on the basis of pigment production (see Table 6.7, p. 172).

For studying the morphology of yeasts, the Dalmau method is recommended. It is performed by using one-fourth or one-third of a cornmeal-Tween 80 agar plate for each organism. Make one streak of a young, actively growing yeast down the center of the area (do not cut the agar); make three or four streaks across the first to dilute the inoculum. Cover with a 22 × 22 mm coverslip and incubate at room temperature, in the dark, for 3 days. Examine by placing the plate, without its lid, on the microscope stage and using the low-power (10x) and high-dry (43x) objectives. The most characteristic morphology (especially the terminal chlamydospores of *Candida albicans*) is often found near the edge of the coverslip.

*C. albicans* should always be included as a control for production of chlamydospores and blastoconidia.

## Dermatophyte Test Medium (DTM)

Specimens from hair, skin, or nails may be inoculated directly onto this medium and incubated at room temperature with the cap of the culture tube loose. Dermatophytes change the color of the medium from yellow to red within 14 days. Care must be taken in specimen collection and interpretation of results, as many contaminants and other fungi increase the number of false-positive changes in color. Dermatophyte test medium does not interfere with macroscopic morphology and microscopic characteristics of the dermatophytes, but it cannot be used to study pigment production because of the intense red color of the indicator.

| | |
|---|---|
| Phytone | 10.0 g |
| Dextrose | 10.0 g |
| Agar | 20.0 g |
| Phenol red solution | 40.0 ml |
| 0.8 M HCl | 6.0 ml |
| Cycloheximide (Upjohn) | 0.5 g |
| Gentamicin sulfate (Schering) | 0.1 g |
| Chlortetracycline HCl (Lederle) | 0.1 g |
| Distilled water | 1,000.0 ml |

## PROCEDURE

1. Dissolve the phytone, dextrose, and agar by boiling in the water.
2. While stirring, add 40 ml of phenol red solution (0.5 g of phenol red dissolved in 15 ml of 0.1 N NaOH made up to 100 ml with distilled water).
3. While stirring, add the 0.8 M HCl.
4. Dissolve cycloheximide in 2 ml of acetone and add to hot medium while stirring.
5. Dissolve gentamicin sulfate in 2 ml of distilled water and add to medium while stirring.
6. Autoclave at 12 lb/in$^2$ for 10 min and cool to approximately 47°C.
7. Dissolve chlortetracycline in 25 ml of sterile distilled water in sterile container and add to medium while stirring.
8. Dispense into sterile 1-oz (~30 ml) screw-cap bottles or screw-cap tubes; slant and cool. The final pH of the medium is 5.5 ± 0.1, and the medium should be yellow in color.
9. Store in refrigerator at 4°C.

# Fermentation Broth for Yeasts

## BROTH

Bromthymol blue ........................ 0.04 g
Powdered yeast extract .............. 4.50 g
Peptone ..................................... 7.50 g
Distilled water .................... 1,000.00 ml

## STOCK CARBOHYDRATE SOLUTIONS

Carbohydrate ................................. 6 g
Distilled water ............................ 100 ml

Filter sterilize through a 0.22-µm-pore-size filter.

## PROCEDURE

1. Dissolve bromthymol blue in 3 ml of 95% ethanol. Add to other ingredients.
2. Dispense 2-ml aliquots into screw-cap tubes.
3. Place Durham tube (mouth down) into each tube of broth.
4. Autoclave at 15 lb/in² for 15 min. Allow to cool.
5. Add 1 ml of each carbohydrate solution to separate tubes of broth. (After the carbohydrates have been added, the broths may be stored for 1 month in the refrigerator.)

Inoculate each of the carbohydrate broths with a pure culture of the organism grown on a sugar-free medium. Be sure that the Durham tube is completely filled with broth before incubating.

Incubate at room temperature for 10–14 days, examining at 48- to 72-h intervals for production of gas (observed in Durham tube). Gas production is the only reliable evidence of carbohydrate fermentation; acid production may simply indicate that the carbohydrate has been assimilated. All fermented carbohydrates will also be assimilated, but many compounds that are assimilated are not necessarily fermented. For identification of yeasts, see Table 4.2 (p. 66) and Table 4.4 (p. 79).

## Gelatin Medium

### FRAZIER PLATE METHOD

The Frazier plate method is the most rapid and reliable test for the ability of microorganisms to decompose gelatin; it is therefore highly recommended over the old conventional butt method.

**Agar**

> Standard method agar (Tryptone Glucose Yeast Agar), BBL
> or
> Tryptone glucose extract agar (Standard Plate Count Agar), Difco .................. 24 g
> Distilled water ........................... 1,000 g

Heat to dissolve, mixing well.
Remove from heat, cool slightly.

Add

> Gelatin .............................................. 4 g

Mix thoroughly until gelatin dissolves.
Autoclave at 15 lb/in$^2$ for 12 min.
Dispense into small petri plates or into screw-cap tubes and allow to solidify as butts to be melted and poured as needed.

**Developer (acid mercuric chloride)**

> Mercuric chloride (HgCl$_2$) .............. 12 g
> Distilled water ................................80 ml
> Concentrated HCl ........................ 16 ml

Prepare in order listed; HgCl$_2$ will dissolve only after HCl is added. Mix well. (An aqueous-saturated solution of ammonium sulfate may also be used as a developer.)

**Procedure**

Inoculate the agar surface in one spot approximately the size of a dime.
Incubate at room temperature until growth is mature.
Flood surface of plate with developer.
Mercuric chloride (or ammonium sulfate) precipitates gelatin, causing the medium to become cloudy where gelatin is intact.
Gelatin decomposition (a positive test) is demonstrated by a clear zone around the colony.
See Table 3.1 (p. 56) and Table 6.3 (p. 129).

## BUTT LIQUEFACTION METHOD

> Brain heart infusion .................... 25 g
> Gelatin ....................................... 120 g
> Distilled water .......................... 1,000 ml

Heat to dissolve ingredients; adjust to pH 7.4–7.6.

Dispense 5- to 8-ml aliquots in 16 × 125 mm screw-cap tubes.

Autoclave at 15 lb/in² for 15 min. Allow to harden as butts.

Inoculate the surface and just below the surface of the medium with the organism to be tested. Incubate tubes at room temperature for 4 weeks.

Examine at weekly intervals for proteolytic activity by placing in refrigerator for 1 h and observing for liquefaction. If the medium solidifies in the refrigerator, proteolysis has not occurred and the tube should be returned to room temperature and retested the following week.

See Table 3.1 (p. 56) and Table 6.3 (p. 129).

---

## Inhibitory Mold Agar (IMA)

Inhibitory mold agar is an enriched medium that contains chloramphenicol but no cycloheximide; bacteria are inhibited while fungi grow well. When specimens are contaminated with bacteria, inhibitory mold agar is used to isolate cycloheximide-sensitive fungi, e.g., *Cryptococcus neoformans*, *Pseudallescheria boydii*, the zygomycetes, many species of *Candida* and *Aspergillus*, and most saprophytic or opportunistic fungi.

Prepare in accordance with manufacturer's instructions (BBL Microbiology Systems, Cockeysville, Md.).

---

## Loeffler Medium

(For testing proteolytic activity of *Cladosporium* species and similar organisms)

The medium may be obtained in dehydrated form or bought commercially prepared from a number of sources.

For use, place a fragment of the fungus on the agar slant, taking care not to place the inoculum on the bottom part of the slant that is usually covered with liquid.

Incubate all tubes at room temperature for 4 weeks.

Examine tubes at weekly intervals for evidence of proteolytic activity, i.e., disintegration of medium.

Usually, saprophytic species of *Cladosporium* are proteolytic, whereas pathogenic species such as *Cladosporium carrionii* and *Xylohypha bantiana* are not (see Table 6.3, p. 129).

## Lysozyme Medium

### BASAL GLYCEROL BROTH

$$
\begin{array}{ll}
\text{Peptone} & 1.0 \text{ g} \\
\text{Beef extract} & 0.6 \text{ g} \\
\text{Glycerol} & 14.0 \text{ ml} \\
\text{Distilled water} & 200.0 \text{ ml}
\end{array}
$$

Combine ingredients; mix well to dissolve.

Pour 95 ml of broth into a separate container.

Dispense the remainder into screw-cap tubes in 5-ml quantities. These will be used as control tubes.

Autoclave broth at 15 lb/in$^2$ for 15 min.

### LYSOZYME BROTH

$$
\begin{array}{ll}
\text{Lysozyme} & 50 \text{ mg} \\
\text{0.01N HCl} & 50 \text{ ml}
\end{array}
$$

Sterilize by filtration.

Aseptically add 5 ml of lysozyme solution to the 95 ml of basal glycerol broth. Mix well. Dispense 5-ml aliquots into sterile screw-cap tubes. Store all tubes in the refrigerator.

Inoculate a tube of control broth (glycerol broth without lysozyme) and a tube of lysozyme broth with the organism to be tested.

Incubate at room temperature until control tube shows good growth. The organism must grow in the control tube for the test to be valid. Growth in the lysozyme broth indicates resistance to the enzyme.

A known *Streptomyces* sp. should be used as a susceptible control organism; i.e., growth must occur in the control tube but not in the lysozyme tube to prove the lysozyme is active.

## Potato Dextrose Agar and Potato Flake Agar

These media are available commercially prepared or in dehydrated form and should be prepared according to manufacturers' instructions. They are often useful in the stimulation of conidia production in fungi and may therefore be most valuable when used in slide cultures.

## Sabouraud Dextrose Agar (SDA)

### EMMONS MODIFICATION

This modification differs from the original formula in that it has an approximately neutral pH and contains only 2% dextrose.

Most mycologists no longer consider it necessary or desirable to use 4% sugar, as in the original formula, and a pH near neutrality has been found to be better for some fungi. The very acid original formula once recommended for suppression of bacterial contaminants can now be replaced by media containing antibiotics.

| | |
|---|---|
| Dextrose | 20 g |
| Peptone | 10 g |
| Agar | 17 g |
| Distilled water | 1,000 ml |

Final pH 6.9.

### ORIGINAL FORMULA

Some workers still prefer the original formula:

| | |
|---|---|
| Dextrose | 40 g |
| Peptone | 10 g |
| Agar | 15 g |
| Distilled water | 1,000 ml |

Final pH is 5.6.

To prepare either of the above formulas, dissolve the ingredients by boiling, dispense in tubes, and autoclave at 15 lb/in² for 10 min.

Allow tubes to cool in slanted position.

Store in refrigerator.

Both formulations of SDA are commercially available in prepared or dehydrated form.

## SDA with Antibiotics

To SDA, while boiling and before autoclaving, add

> Cycloheximide (Upjohn Co.) ........ 500 mg
> Chloramphenicol
>   (Parke-Davis & Co.) .................. 50 mg

Dissolve the cycloheximide in 10 ml of acetone and add it to the boiling medium. Mix well.

Dissolve the chloramphenicol in 10 ml of 95% ethanol and add to boiling medium. Remove from heat and mix well.

Dispense in tubes; autoclave at 15 lb/in$^2$ for 10 min.

Allow to cool in slanted position.

Store in refrigerator.

Comparable media commercially available include Mycosel Agar (BBL, Cockeysville, Md.) and Mycobiotic Agar (Difco Laboratories, Detroit, Mich.).

## SDA with 15% NaCl

Testing for tolerance to 15% sodium chloride (NaCl) can be valuable for identifying some dematiaceous (black) fungi.

> SDA ............................................ 500 ml
> NaCl ........................................... 75 g

Heat to dissolve.

Dispense in tubes; autoclave at 15 lb/in$^2$ for 10 min.

Allow to solidify as butts to be melted and slanted as needed.

Place a pinpoint inoculum of the organism to be tested on a slant of the agar. Incubate at room temperature.

The organism is considered to be strongly inhibited if its colony diameter is less than 2 mm at 21 days. If the colony surpasses 2 mm, the organism is considered tolerant of 15% NaCl.

## Sabouraud Dextrose Broth

> Dextrose ..................................... 20 mg
> Peptone ...................................... 10 mg
> Distilled water ........................ 1,000 ml

Final pH is 5.7.

Dissolve ingredients; dispense into tubes.

Autoclave (15 lb/in$^2$) for 10 min.

Noting the manner in which yeasts grow in this broth can assist in their identification (see Table 4.1, p. 64, and Table 4.2, p. 66). Sabouraud dextrose broth is also used for the detection of fungal contaminants in pharmaceutical products.

## Starch Hydrolysis Agar
(For aerobic actinomycetes and dematiaceous fungi)

> Nutrient agar ............................... 23 g
> Potato starch .............................. 10 g
> Demineralized water .............. 1,000 ml

Dissolve agar in 500 ml of water by boiling.
Dissolve starch in 250 ml of water by boiling.
Combine and add 250 ml of water.
Dispense into screw-cap tubes.
Autoclave (15 lb/in²) for 30 min.
Allow to cool as butts; melt down and pour into petri plates as needed.

## PROCEDURE
Inoculate a 10-mm round area of agar heavily with a pure culture of the organism to be tested. Incubate at optimal growth temperature until good growth occurs.

Flood the area around the growth with Gram iodine.

Starch hydrolysis is demonstrated by a colorless (complete hydrolysis) or red (partial hydrolysis) area around the growth. Unhydrolyzed starch in the medium will produce a deep blue to purple color in the presence of iodine (see Table 3.1, p. 56).

## Trichophyton Agars

(Nutritional requirement tests for the differentiation of *Trichophyton* spp.)

These agars are available commercially prepared or in dehydrated form. Rehydration is performed according to manufacturer's instructions.

The set of seven media tests the growth factor requirements of the species of *Trichophyton*. They are often helpful in differentiating the species. Their composition is as follows:

No. 1. Casein agar base (vitamin free)

No. 2. Casein agar base plus inositol

No. 3. Casein agar base plus inositol and thiamine

No. 4. Casein agar base plus thiamine

No. 5. Casein agar base plus nicotinic acid

No. 6. Ammonium nitrate agar base

No. 7. Ammonium nitrate agar base plus histidine

### INOCULATION OF MEDIA

The center of a slant of each medium is inoculated with a small and equal size fragment of pure culture grown on SDA with or without antibiotics. It is important that the culture be free of bacteria, for many bacteria synthesize vitamins which may invalidate the test. Care must also be taken not to transfer any of the SDA with the organism, as this may supply carryover nutrients and cause false reactions.

A homogeneous suspension of fuzzy or granular colonies should be made in sterile saline or water. Two drops of the suspension is placed on each slant of medium. This method of inoculation dilutes possible carryover nutrients and ensures that each slant receives an equal inoculum.

Tubes are incubated at room temperature for 2 weeks and examined periodically for growth. The tube that shows maximum growth is recorded as 4 +. Other tubes are graded by comparison.

For interpretation of results, see Table 6.7 (p. 172) and Table 6.8 (p. 180).

## Tyrosine or Xanthine Agar

(For differentiation of aerobic actinomycetes and characterization of *Exophiala*, *Wangiella*, and *Phaeoannellomyces* spp.)

| | |
|---|---|
| Nutrient agar | 23 g |
| Tyrosine | 5 g |
| (or xanthine | 4 g) |
| Distilled water | 1,000 ml |

Dissolve agar in the distilled water by boiling (swirl frequently).

Add tyrosine or xanthine, taking care to distribute the crystals evenly throughout the agar.

Adjust to pH 7.0; autoclave at 15 lb/in² for 15 min.

If the agar is too hot when poured, the time required for solidification will be long enough to permit settling out of the tyrosine or xanthine granules. To avoid this, the medium should be allowed to cool to 45–48°C before pouring and the flask should be mixed well while the plates are poured to ensure an even distribution of the crystals. If the medium is to be stored for a long period, pour well-mixed medium, with evenly distributed crystals, into tubes. Allow to solidify as butts and refrigerate. When needed, place tubes of agar in boiling water bath to melt, cool to 45–48°C, mix well to resuspend crystals, and pour into petri plates.

Heavily inoculate an area of agar 10 mm in diameter with a pure culture. Incubate at room temperature or at 35–37°C for 2–3 weeks. Examine every 3 or 4 days for clearing of the medium around or directly beneath the colony, which indicates hydrolysis.

For interpretation of results, see Table 3.1 (p. 56) and Table 6.5 (p. 138).

## Urea Agar

> **A.** Urea agar base (Christensen) ........ 29 g
> Distilled water ........................... 100 ml

Dissolve the powder in the water and sterilize by filtration.

> **B.** Agar ............................................. 15 g
> Distilled water ........................... 900 ml

Dissolve agar in the water and sterilize by autoclaving at 15 lb/in² for 15 min.
Cool the agar to approximately 50°C.
Add the 100 ml of sterile urea agar base.
Mix well; dispense aseptically into sterile tubes.
Allow to cool in slanted position to form butt about 1 in. (2.5 cm) deep and slant approximately 1.5 in. (3.8 cm) long.

Urease-positive organisms produce an alkaline reaction indicated by a pink-red color.

This medium is used for the differentiation of the yeastlike fungi and also in the identification of some *Trichophyton* species and aerobic actinomycetes. It is commercially available in prepared or dehydrated form.

## Yeast Extract-Phosphate Agar with Ammonia

(For isolation of *Histoplasma capsulatum* and *Blastomyces dermatitidis* from contaminated specimens)

### PHOSPHATE BUFFER

| | |
|---|---:|
| $Na_2HPO_4$ | 4 g |
| $KH_2PO_4$ | 6 g |
| Distilled water | 30 ml |

Mix well to dissolve; adjust pH to 6.0 with 1 N HCl or 1 N NaOH.

### YEAST EXTRACT SOLUTION

| | |
|---|---:|
| Yeast extract | 1 g |
| Agar | 20 g |
| Chloramphenicol (optional) | 50 mg |
| Distilled water | 1,000 ml |

Mix; bring to boil while stirring frequently.

Add 2 ml of phosphate buffer to the liter of yeast extract solution. Mix well.
Dispense 17–18 ml into screw-cap tubes.
Autoclave at 15 lb/in$^2$ for 15 min.

As needed, melt and pour two tubes of medium (35 ml) into a sterile petri plate. Spread approximately 0.5 ml of specimen over surface of solidified agar. Place one drop (0.05 ml) of concentrated $NH_4OH$ off center on the agar surface. Allow it to diffuse. Incubate at 25–30°C. The diffusing $NH_4OH$ inhibits bacteria, yeasts, and many molds while allowing slow growing dimorphic fungi to grow.

# Glossary

**Abscess:**  Localized collection of pus in cavity formed by dissolution of tissue.

**Aerial hyphae:**  Hyphae above the agar surface.

**Aerobic:**  Able to grow in the presence of atmospheric oxygen.

**Anaerobic:**  Able to grow in the absence of free or atmospheric oxygen.

**Annellide:**  A cell that produces and extrudes conidia; the tip tapers, lengthens, and acquires a ring of cell wall material as each conidium is released; oil immersion magnification may be required to see the rings.

**Apex (pl. *apices*):**  The tip.

**Apophysis:**  The swelling of a sporangiophore immediately below the columella.

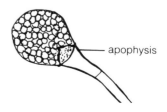

apophysis

**Arthroconidium:** An asexual spore formed by the breaking up of a hypha at the point of septation. The resulting cell may be rectangular or barrel shaped and thick or thin walled, depending on the genus.

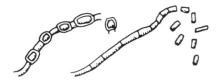

**Ascospore:** A sexual spore produced in a sac-like structure known as an *ascus*.

**Ascus (pl. *asci*):** A round or elongate sac-like structure containing usually two to eight ascospores. The asci are often formed within a fruiting body, such as a cleistothecium or perithecium.

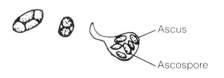

Ascus

Ascospore

**Asexual:** Reproduction in an organism by division or redistribution of nuclei, but without nuclear fusion, i.e., not by the union of two nuclei. Also known as *imperfect state*.

**Assimilation:** The ability to use a carbon or nitrogen source for growth.

**Basidiospore:** A sexual spore formed on a structure known as a *basidium*. Characteristic of the class Basidiomycetes.

**Biseriate:** With reference to the genus *Aspergillus*, phialide is supported by a metula as opposed to a uniseriate phialide which forms directly on the vesicle. (See *Uniseriate*.)

**Blastoconidium:** A conidium formed by budding along a hypha, pseudohypha, or single cell, as in the yeasts.

**Budding:** A process of asexual reproduction in which the new cell develops as a smaller outgrowth from the older parent cell. Characteristic of yeasts or yeastlike fungi.

**Capsule:** A colorless, transparent, mucopolysaccharide sheath on the wall of a cell.

**Chlamydoconidium:** An enlarged, rounded conidium that is thick walled and contains stored food, enabling it to function as a survival propagule. It may be located at the end of the hypha (ter-

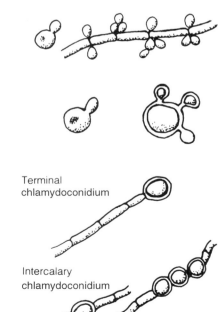

Terminal
chlamydoconidium

Intercalary
chlamydoconidium

minal) or inserted along the hypha (intercalary), singly or in chains. Characteristically, it is greater in diameter than the hypha on which it is borne. Unlike other conidia, it does not readily separate from the hypha.

**Chlamydospore:** The misnomer applied to the thick-walled vesicle formed by *Candida albicans*. It neither germinates nor produces conidia when mature.

**Chloramphenicol:** An antibiotic (proprietary name, Chloromycetin; Parke-Davis & Co., Detroit, Mich.) produced by *Streptomyces venezuelae*, but usually prepared synthetically. It is a useful additive to mycology media, as it inhibits the growth of many bacteria that might contaminate the cultures.

**Clamp connection:** A specialized bridge over a hyphal septum in the Basidiomycetes. During the formation of a new cell, it allows postmitosis nuclear migration.

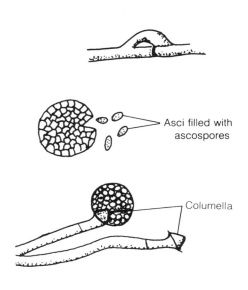

Asci filled with ascospores

**Cleistothecium:** A large, fairly round, closed, many-celled structure in which asci and ascospores are formed and held until the structure bursts.

Columella

**Columella:** The enlarged, dome-shaped tip of a sporangiophore that extends into the sporangium. Often the sporangium bursts, leaving the columella bare and readily visible upon microscopic examination.

**Conidiogenous cell:** The cell that produces the conidia.

**Conidiophore:** A specialized hyphal structure that serves as a stalk on which conidia are formed. The shape and arrangement of the conidiophores and the conidia are generally characteristic of a genus. The suffix, -*phore*, means "carrying" and is added to the word that denotes what it is carrying, e.g., conidiophores bear conidia and sporangiophores bear sporangia.

**Conidium (pl. *conidia*):** Asexual propagule that forms on the side or the end of the hypha or conidiophore. It may consist of one or more cells, and the size, shape, and arrangement in groups are generally characteristic of the organism. It is always borne externally, i.e., not enclosed within a sac-like structure such as a sporangium. If a fungus produces two types of conidia, those that are small and usually single celled are re-

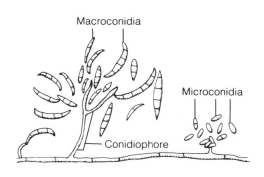

Macroconidia

Microconidia

Conidiophore

ferred to as *microconidia*, whereas the larger *macroconidia* are usually segmented into two or more cells.

**Cutaneous:**  Pertaining to the skin.

**Cycloheximide:**  An antibiotic (proprietary name, Actidione; Upjohn Co., Kalamazoo, Mich.) used in selective mycology media to inhibit the growth of saprophytic fungi. Because it is also known to inhibit some pathogenic fungi, it must be used in conjunction with a medium without antibiotics.

**Dematiaceous:**  Having structures that are brown to black; this is due to a melanotic pigment in the cell walls.

**Denticle:**  Short, narrow projection bearing a conidium.

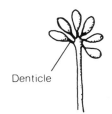
Denticle

**Dermatophyte:**  A fungus belonging to the genus *Trichophyton, Microsporum,* or *Epidermophyton* with the ability to obtain nutrients from keratin and infect skin, hair, or nails of humans or animals.

**Dichotomous:**  Branching of hyphae into two equal branches that are each equal in diameter to the hypha from which they originated.

**Dimorphic:**  Having two distinct morphological forms. In this guide, it refers to temperature-dependent changes in the organism on artificial culture media, i.e., fungi having a mold phase when cultured at 25–30°C and a yeast phase when cultured at 35–37°C.

**Favic chandeliers:**  Terminal hyphal branches that are irregular, broad, and antler-like in appearance. Especially characteristic of *Trichophyton schoenleini.*

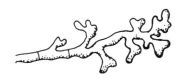

**Filamentous:**  Long, cylindrical, and threadlike; hyphae forming.

**Floccose:**  Cottony; like raw, fuzzy cotton.

**Foot cell:**  The base of the conidiophore, where it merges with the hyphae, giving the impression of a foot; typically seen in *Aspergillus* spp.

**Fragmentation:**  Breaking of the hyphae into pieces, each of which is capable of forming a new organism. Arthroconidia are formed in this manner.

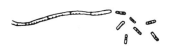

**Fungus (pl. *fungi*):**  An organism that is either filamentous or unicellular and lacks chlorophyll. It has a true nucleus enclosed in a membrane and chitin in the cell wall.

**Fusiform:**   Spindle shaped, i.e., being wider in the middle and narrowing toward the ends.

**Geniculate:**   Bent like a knee.

**Germ tube:**   A tubelike outgrowth from a conidium or spore; the beginning of a hypha.

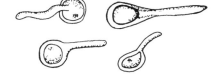

**Glabrous:**   Smooth; without or almost without aerial hyphae.

**Hilum (pl. *hila*):**   scar of attachment; it appears at the point(s) where the conidium was formerly attached to the conidiophore and/or another conidium.

**Host:**   The animal or plant that supports a parasite.

**Hülle cells:**   Thickened large sterile cells with a small lumen; they are associated with cleistothecia produced by the sexual stage of some *Aspergillus* spp.

**Hyaline:**   Clear, transparent, colorless.

**Hypha (pl. *hyphae*):**   A filamentous structure of a fungus. Many together compose the mycelium.

**Hyphomycete:**   An asexual fungus that produces mycelium that may be colorless (hyaline) or darkly pigmented (dematiaceous).

**Inflammation:**   A local protective response of the body; characterized by redness, pain, heat, and swelling.

**Intercalary:**   Situated along the hypha, not at its end.

**Intracellular:**   Within cells.

**Keratin:**   A scleroprotein containing large amounts of sulfur, such as cystine; the primary component of skin, hair, and nails.

**Keratitis:**   Inflammation of the cornea of the eye.

**Macroconidium (pl. *macroconidia*):**   The larger of two types of conidia in a fungus that produces both large and small conidia; may be single celled, but usually is multicelled. (See *Conidium.*)

**Metula (pl. *metulae*):**   The structure below the phialides of some *Aspergillus* and *Penicillium* spp.

**Microconidium (pl. *microconidia*):**   The smaller of two types of conidia in a fungus that produces both large and small conidia; usually single celled and round, ovoid, pear shaped, or club shaped. (See *Conidium.*)

**Mold:**   A filamentous fungus composed of filaments that generally form a colony that may be either fuzzy, powdery, woolly, velvety, or relatively smooth.

**Monomorphic:**   In this guide, refers to fungi having the same type of morphology in culture at both 25–30°C and 35–37°C (i.e., if growth occurs at both temperature ranges; some saprophytes are inhibited at 35–37°C).

**Muriform:** Having transverse and longitudinal septations.

**Mycelium (pl. *mycelia*):** A mat of intertwined hyphae that constitutes the colony surface of a mold.

**Mycetoma:** A localized, chronic cutaneous or subcutaneous infection classically characterized by draining sinuses, granules, and swelling.

**Mycology:** The study of fungi and their biology.

**Mycosis (pl. *mycoses*):** A disease caused by a fungus.

**Nodular body:** A round knot-like structure formed by intertwined hyphae; seen especially in some dermatophytes.

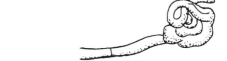

**Ostiole:** A mouth or opening.

**Pathogen:** Any disease-producing microorganism.

**Pectinate:** Resembling a comb.

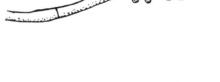

**Pellicle:** A firm or buttonlike mass formed on liquid medium by some fungi.

**Perithecium (pl. *perithecia*):** A large, round or pear-shaped structure usually having a small rounded opening (which differentiates it from a cleistothecium; the opening is called an *ostiole*) and containing asci and ascospores.

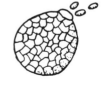

**Phaeo:** A prefix meaning dark (brownish or blackish).

**Phaeohyphomycosis:** A subcutaneous or systemic disease caused by a variety of black fungi that develop in tissue as dark hyphae and/or yeastlike cells.

**Phialide:** A cell that produces and extrudes conidia without tapering or increasing in length with each new conidium produced. It is usually shaped like a flask, vase, or tenpin.

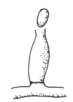

**Pleomorphism:** The occurrence of two or more forms in the life cycle of an organism. Also refers to the occurrence of a form of dermatophyte that ceases to produce conidia (becomes sterile).

**Propagule:** A unit that can give rise to another organism.

**Pseudohypha:** Chain of cells formed by budding which, when elongated, resembles a true hypha; differs from true hyphae by being constricted at the septa, forming branches that begin with a septation, and having terminal cells smaller than the other cells.

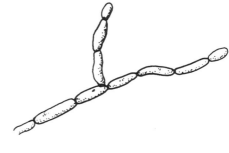

**Pycnidium (pl. _pycnidia_):** A large, round or flask-shaped fruiting body containing conidia. Pycnidia usually have an opening (an ostiole).

**Pyriform:** Pear shaped.

**Racquet hypha:** A hypha with club-shaped cells, the larger end of one cell being attached to the smaller end of an adjacent cell.

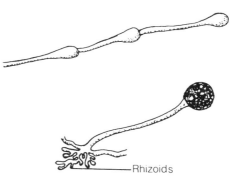

**Rhizoid:** Rootlike, branched hypha extending into the medium.

Rhizoids

**Ringworm:** Superficial skin disease caused by dermatophytes. Term derived from the ring-like, circular form of the lesions and from the belief that these infections were caused by worm-like organisms. The current accepted term is _tinea._

**Saprobe/Saprophyte:** An organism that uses dead organic matter as a source of nutrients.

**Septate:** Having cross walls.

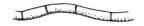

**Sexual state:** The portion of the life cycle in which the organism reproduces by the union of two nuclei. Also known as the _perfect state._

**Spherule:** Large, round, thick-walled structure containing spores; characteristic of _Coccidioides immitis_ in infected host material under direct microscopic examination. Spherules do not grow on routine artificial mycology media.

**Spiral hypha:** Hypha forming coiled or corkscrewlike turns.

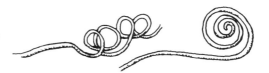

**Sporangiophore:** A specialized hyphal branch or stalk bearing a sporangium.

**Sporangiospore:** An asexual spore produced in a sporangium.

**Sporangium (pl. *sporangia*):** A closed sac-like structure in which asexual spores (sporangiospores) are formed by cleavage.

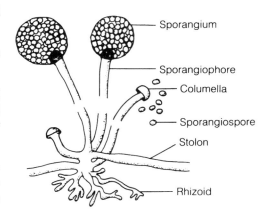

**Spore:** Propagule that develops by sexual reproduction (ascospore, basidiospore, zygospore) or by asexual means within a sporangium (sporangiospore). Those most commonly seen in the clinical laboratory are usually enclosed in a sac-like structure (as opposed to conidia which are free, not enclosed).

**Sterigmata:** Term formerly used to denote phialides of *Aspergillus* and other genera. More accurately refers to denticles produced by Basidiomycetes.

**Stolon:** A horizontal hypha, or runner, that grows along the surface of the medium, often bearing rhizoids that penetrate the medium and sporangiophores that ascend into the air.

**Subcutaneous:** Situated or occurring directly under the skin.

**Suppurative:** Producing pus.

**Sympodial growth:** Conidiogenous structure that continues to increase in length by forming a new growing point just below each new terminal conidium, often resulting in a geniculate (bent) appearance.

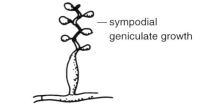

**Thallus:** The vegetative body of a fungus.

**Terminal:** At the end.

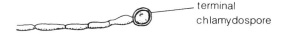

**Truncate:** Cut off sharply; ending abruptly with a flattened edge.

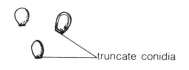

**Tuberculate:** Having knoblike projections.

**Uniseriate:** With reference to the genus *Aspergillus*, phialide forms directly on the vesicle; a biseriate phialide is supported by a metula.

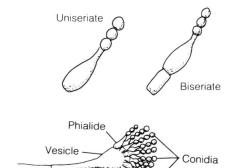

**Vesicle:** Enlarged structure at the end of a conidiophore or sporangiophore. In *Aspergillus* spp. it bears the phialides, which in turn bear the conidia.

**Whorl:** A group of cells radiating from a common point.

**Yeastlike colony:** A soft, pasty, smooth colony; usually no filamentous (fuzzy) growth can be observed macroscopically.

# Bibliography

## Suggested for Further Information

**Barron, G. L. 1977.** *The Genera of Hyphomycetes from Soil.* Robert E. Krieger Publishing Co., Huntington, N.Y.

**Blinkhorn, R. J., D. Adelstein, and P. J. Spagnuolo. 1989.** Emergence of a new opportunistic pathogen, *Candida lusitaniae. J. Clin. Microbiol.* **27:**236–240.

**Chandler, F. W., and J. C. Watts. 1987.** *Pathologic Diagnosis of Fungal Infections.* American Society of Clinical Pathology Press, Chicago.

**Dixon, D. M., and A. Polak-Wyss. 1991.** The medically important dematiaceous fungi and their identification. *Mycoses* **34:**1–18.

**Dixon, D. M., and I. F. Salkin. 1986.** Morphologic and physiologic studies of three dematiaceous pathogens. *J. Clin. Microbiol.* **24:**12–15.

**Evans, E. G. V., and M. D. Richardson (ed.). 1989.** *Medical Mycology; a Practical Approach.* IRL Press, Oxford.

**Hilmarsdottir, I., J. L. Meynard, O. Rogeaux, G. Guermonprez, A. Datry, C. Katlama, G. Brücker, A. Coutellier, M. Danis, and M. Gentilini. 1993.** Disseminated *Penicillium marneffei* infection associated with human immunodeficiency virus: a report of two cases and a review of 35 published cases. *J. Acquired Immune Defic. Syndr.* **6:**466–471.

**Ibrahim-Granet, O., and C. de Bievere. 1984.** Study of the conidial development and cleistothecium-like structure of some strains of *Fonsecaea pedrosoi. Mycopathologia* **84:**181–186.

**Isenberg, H. D. (ed.). 1992.** *Clinical Microbiology Procedures Handbook.* American Society for Microbiology, Washington, D.C.

**Kane, J., R. Summerbell, L. Sigler, S. Krajden, and G. Land.** *Laboratory Handbook of Dermatophytes*, in press. Star Publishing Co., Belmont, Calif.

**Kemna, M. E., R. C. Neri, R. Ali, and I. F. Salkin. 1994.** *Cokeromyces recurvatus*, a mucoraceous zygomycete rarely isolated in clinical laboratories. *J. Clin. Microbiol.* **32:**843–845.

**Koneman, E. W., and G. D. Roberts. 1991.** Mycotic disease, p. 1104–1110. *In* J. B. Henry (ed.), *Clinical Diagnosis and Management by Laboratory Methods.* W.B. Saunders Co., Philadelphia.

**Kreger-van Rij, N. J. W. (ed.). 1984.** *The Yeasts*, 3rd ed. Elsevier Science Publishers, Amsterdam.

**Kwon-Chung, K. J., and J. E. Bennett. 1992.** *Medical Mycology.* Lea and Febiger, Philadelphia.

**Levenson, D., M. A. Pfaller, M. A. Smith, R. Hollis, T. Gerarden, C. B. Tucci, and H. D. Isenberg. 1991.** *Candida zeylanoides*: an opportunistic yeast. *J. Clin. Microbiol.* **29:**1689–1692.

**Marcon, M. J., and D. A. Powell. 1992.** Human infections due to *Malassezia* spp. *Clin. Microbiol. Rev.* **5:**101–119.

**McGinnis, M. R. 1980.** *Laboratory Handbook of Medical Mycology.* Academic Press, New York.

**McGinnis, M. R. 1994.** *Penicillium marneffei*, dimorphic fungus of increasing importance. *Clin. Microbiol. Newsl.* **16:**29–31.

**McGinnis, M. R., M. G. Rinaldi, and R. E. Winn. 1986.** Emerging agents of phaeohyphomycosis: pathogenic species of *Bipolaris* and *Exserohilum. J. Clin. Microbiol.* **24:**250–259.

**McGough, D. A., A. W. Fothergill, and M. G. Rinaldi. 1990.** *Cokeromyces recurvatus* Poitras, a distinctive zygomycete and potential pathogen: criteria for identification. *Clin. Microbiol. Newsl.* **12:**113–117.

**McNeil, M. M., and J. M. Brown. 1994.** The medically important aerobic actinomycetes: epidemiology and microbiology. *Clin. Microbiol. Rev.* **7:**357–417.

**Misra, P. C., K. J. Srivastava, and K. Lata. 1979.** *Apophysomyces*, a new genus of the Mucorales. *Mycotaxon* **8:**377–382.

**Murray, P. R., E. J. Baron, M. A. Pfaller, F. C. Tenover, and R. H. Yolken (ed.). 1995.** *Manual of Clinical Microbiology*, 6th ed. American Society for Microbiology, Washington, D.C.

**Polacheck, I., I. F. Salkin, R. Kitzes-Cohen, and R. Raz. 1992.** Endocarditis caused by *Blastoschizomyces capitatus* and taxonomic review of the genus. *J. Clin. Microbiol.* **30:**2318–2322.

**Raper, K. B., and D. L. Fennell. 1973.** *The Genus Aspergillus.* Robert E. Krieger Publishing Co., Huntington, N.Y.

**Rebell, G., and D. Taplin. 1970.** *Dermatophytes, Their Recognition and Identification,* 2nd ed. University of Miami Press, Coral Gables, Fla.

**Rippon, J. W. 1988.** *Medical Mycology: the Pathogenic Fungi and the Pathogenic Actinomycetes,* 3rd ed. W.B. Saunders Company, Philadelphia.

**Salkin, I. F., M. A. Gordon, W. A. Samsonoff, and C. L. Reider. 1985a.** *Blastoschizomyces capitatus,* a new combination. *Mycotaxon* **22:**373–380.

**Saubolle, M. A., and J. Sutton. 1994.** Coccidioidomycosis: centennial year on the North American continent. *Clin. Microbiol. Newsl.* **16:**137–144.

**Walsh, T. J., G. Renshaw, J. Andrews, J. Kwon-Chung, R. C. Cunnion, H. I. Pass, J. Taubenberger, W. Wilson, and P. A. Pizzo. 1994.** Invasive zygomycosis due to *Conidiobolus incongruus. Clin. Infect. Dis.* **19:**423–430.

**Wentworth, B. B. (ed.). 1988.** *Diagnostic Procedures for Mycotic and Parasitic Infections,* 7th ed. American Public Health Association, Washington, D.C.

**Wilson, J. W., and O. A. Plunkett. 1970.** *The Fungous Diseases of Man.* University of California Press, Berkeley.

## Additional References

**Adams, E. D., and B. H. Cooper. 1974.** Evaluation of a modified Wickerham medium for identifying medically important yeasts. *Am. J. Med. Technol.* **40:**377–388.

**Baker, J. G., H. L. Nadler, P. Forgacs, and S. R. Kurtz. 1984.** *Candida lusitaniae*: a new opportunistic pathogen of the urinary tract. *Diagn. Microbiol. Infect. Dis.* **2:**145–149.

**Baker, J. G., I. F. Salkin, D. H. Pincus, and R. F. D'Amato. 1981.** *Candida paratropicalis,* a new species of *Candida. Mycotaxon* **13:**115–119.

**Barnett, J. A., R. W. Payne, and D. Yarrow. 1991.** *Yeasts: Characteristics and Identification,* 2nd ed. Cambridge University Press, New York.

**Bottone, E. J., I. Weitzman, and B. A. Hanna. 1979.** *Rhizopus rhizopodiformis*: emerging etiological agent of mucormycosis. *J. Clin. Microbiol.* **9:**530–537.

**Bottone, E. J., and G. P. Wormser. 1985.** Capsule-deficient cryptococci in AIDS. *Lancet* **ii:**553.

**Carmichael, J. W. 1962.** *Chrysosporium* and some other alleuriosporic hyphomycetes. *Can. J. Botany* **40:**1137–1173.

**Carmichael, J. W., W. B. Kendrick, I. L. Conners, and L. Sigler. 1980.** *Genera of Hyphomycetes.* University of Alberta Press, Alberta, Canada.

**Crozier, W. J. 1993.** Two cases of onychomycosis due to *Candida zeylanoides*. *Aust. J. Dermatol.* **34:**23–25.

**de Hoog, G. S. 1983.** On the potentially pathogenic dematiaceous hyphomycetes, p. 149–217. *In* D. H. Howard (ed.), *Fungi Pathogenic for Humans and Animals*, Part A. Marcel Dekker, New York.

**Fincher, R.-M. E., J. F. Fisher, R. D. Lovell, C. L. Newman, A. Espinel-Ingroff, and H. J. Shadomy. 1991.** Infection due to the fungus *Acremonium (Cephalosporium)*. *Medicine* **70:**398–409.

**Guého, E., M. T. Smith, G. S. deHoog, G. Billon-Grand, R. Christen, and W. H. Batenburg-van der Vegte. 1992.** Contributions to a revision of the genus *Trichosporon*. *Antonie Leeuwenhoek* **61:**289–316.

**Huber, W. M., and S. M. Caplin. 1947.** Simple and plastic mount for permanent preservation of fungi and small arthropods. *Arch. Dermatol. Syphilol.* **56:**763–765.

**Jones, J. M. 1990.** Laboratory diagnosis of invasive candidiasis. *Clin. Microbiol. Rev.* **3:**32–45.

**Kemna, M. E., M. Weinberger, L. Sigler, R. Zeltser, I. Polacheck, and I. F. Salkin. 1994.** A primary oral blastomycosis-like infection in Israel, abstr. F-75, p. 601. *Abstr. 94th Gen. Meet. Am. Soc. Microbiol. 1994.* American Society for Microbiology, Washington, D.C.

**Larone, D. H. 1989.** The identification of dematiaceous fungi. *Clin. Microbiol. Newsl.* **11:**145–150.

**Larone, D., and I. Beaty. 1988.** Evaluation and modification of tests for phenoloxidase activity in *Cryptococcus neoformans*, abstr. F-111, p. 410. *Abstr. 88th Annu. Meet. Am. Soc. Microbiol. 1988.* American Society for Microbiology, Washington, D.C.

**Liao, W. Q., Z. G. Li, M. Guo, and J. Z. Zhang. 1993.** *Candida zeylanoides* causing candidiasis as tinea cruris. *Chin. Med. J.* **106:**542–545.

**Libertin, C. R., W. R. Wilson, and G. D. Roberts. 1985.** *Candida lusitaniae*: an opportunistic pathogen. *Diagn. Microbiol. Infect. Dis.* **3:**69–71.

**Mahan, C. T., and G. E. Sale. 1978.** Rapid methenamine silver stain for *Pneumocystis* and fungi. *Arch. Pathol. Lab. Med.* **102:**351–352.

**Martino, P., M. Venditti, A. Micozzi, G. Morace, L. Polonelli, M. P. Mantovani, M. C. Petti, V. L. Burgio, C. Santini, P. Serra, and F. Mandelli. 1990.** *Blastoschizomyces capitis*: an emerging cause of invasive fungal disease in leukemia patients. *Rev. Infect. Dis.* **12:**570–582.

**McGinnis, M. R. 1983.** Chromoblastomycosis and phaeohyphomycosis: new concepts, diagnosis, and mycology. *J. Am. Acad. Dermatol.* **8:**1–16.

**McGinnis, M. R., L. Ajello, and W. A. Schell. 1985.** Mycotic diseases: a proposed nomenclature. *Int. J. Dermatol.* **24:**9–15.

**Mok, W. Y. 1982.** Nature and identification of *Exophiala werneckii*. *J. Clin. Microbiol.* **16:**976–978.

**Morris, J. T., M. Beckius, and C. K. McAllister. 1991.** *Sporobolomyces* infection in an AIDS patient. *J. Infect. Dis.* **164:**623–624.

**Nahass, G. T., S. P. Rosenberg, C. L. Leonardi, and N. S. Penneys. 1993.** Disseminated infection with *Trichosporon beigelii.* Report of a case and review of the cutaneous and histologic manifestations. *Arch. Dermatol.* **129:**1020–1023.

**Padhye, A. A., and L. Ajello. 1988.** Simple method of inducing sporulation by *Apophysomyces elegans* and *Saksenaea vasiformis. J. Clin. Microbiol.* **26:**1861–1863.

**Padhye, A. A., J. G. Baker, and R. F. D'Amato. 1979.** Rapid identification of *Prototheca* species by the API 20C system. *J. Clin. Microbiol.* **10:**579–82.

**Pasarell, L., M. E. Kemna, M. R. McGinnis, and I. F. Salkin. 1993.** Mycetoma caused by *Phialophora verrucosa*, abstr. F-31, p. 532. *Abstr. 93rd Gen. Meet. Am. Soc. Microbiol. 1993.* American Society for Microbiology, Washington, D.C.

**Roberts, G. D. 1994.** Laboratory methods in basic mycology, p. 689–775. *In* E. J. Baron, L. R. Peterson, and S. M. Finegold, *Bailey & Scott's Diagnostic Microbiology.* Mosby, St. Louis.

**Salkin, I. F., D. M. Dixon, M. E. Kemna, P. J. Danneman, and J. W. Griffith. 1990.** Fatal encephalitis caused by *Dactylaria constrica* var. *gallopava* in a snowy owl chick (*Nyctea scandiaca*). *J. Clin. Microbiol.* **28:**2845–2847.

**Salkin, I. F., G. E. Hollick, N. J. Hurd, and M. E. Kemna. 1985b.** Evaluation of human hair sources for the in vitro hair perforation test. *J. Clin. Microbiol.* **22:**1048–1049.

**Scholer, H. J., E. Muller, and M. A. A. Schipper. 1983.** Mucorales, p. 9–59. *In* D. H. Howard (ed.), *Fungi Pathogenic for Humans and Animals*, part A. Marcel Dekker, New York.

**Walsh, T. J., G. P. Melcher, M. G. Rinaldi, J. Lecciones, D. A. McGough, P. Kelly, J. Lee, D. Callender, M. Rubin, and P. A. Pizzo. 1990.** *Trichosporon beigelii*, an emerging pathogen resistant to amphotericin B. *J. Clin. Microbiol.* **28:**1616–1622.

**Wang, C. J. K., and R. A. Zabel (ed.). 1990.** *Identification Manual for Fungi from Utility Poles in the Eastern United States.* American Type Culture Collection, Rockville, Md.

# Index